The Apple Cider Vinegar Miracle

81 Ways to Naturally Cleanse

Your Body & House and More!

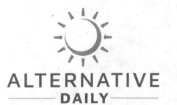

ALTERNATIVE
DAILY

This page intentionally left blank.

The Alternative Daily

This page intentionally left blank.

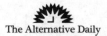

Table of Contents

The Alternative Daily

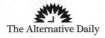

This page intentionally left blank.

Preface

"A man may esteem himself happy when that which is his food is also his medicine."~Henry David Thoreau

Apple cider vinegar (ACV) falls right in line with garlic as being one of the most talked-about natural remedies in folk medicine. Perhaps you remember it as your grandmother's favorite "go-to" in times of need, whether it was for an upset stomach, a cough or to ease dry and chapped skin.

Introduced to the United States in the 1950's by D.C. Jarvis, author of *Folk Medicine: A Vermont Doctor's Guide to Good Health*, ACV is finally being embraced as a dietary supplement worthy of attention.

Traditional uses of ACV are vast. To name just a few, it has been used to ease digestion, aid in flu prevention, reduce inflammation, regulate pH balance, alleviate allergy symptoms, ease nausea and heartburn, as a staple in detox regimens, and for a number of skin conditions, including reducing acne and smoothing wrinkles.

Known in some circles as "Mother Nature's Perfect Miracle Food," unpasteurized and organic ACV truly has much to offer, despite the fact that it has survived a litany of malicious sneers by those who only consider a natural substance to be a credible remedy if it has been studied over and over again, and produced "viable" scientific evidence to earn its merit.

The Alternative Daily

It's just not like that with ACV. Ask anyone why it works for them and they may tell you: "Not sure, it just does." Now, that is not to say that there isn't evidence for its potency and far-reaching applicability to a plethora of conditions - that exists as well, it just doesn't 'stick out'.

Much of what you read on the Internet and in other books does little to substantiate the use of ACV, but only begs one to try. Don't let this fool you, there is actually a great deal of science behind just how and why ACV seems to be a "cure-all" for so many things. Yes, there is also hype and confusion around what works and what doesn't work, but all one has to do is look just a little below the surface to uncover the amazing attributes of apples allowed to slowly ferment.

This book is a marriage of what exists both scientifically and anecdotally, an attempt to satisfy you, the ever curious seeker of alternative practices. It is designed to shed light on effective and economical options to rid your body and home of toxins, to let you know that safer options exist for you and your family, and to reaffirm that sometimes, what seems too simple to be true may be just what we need.

Remember, we are conditioned to believe that natural cures don't work, and we must put our faith in dangerous pharmaceuticals if we wish to find relief. Breaking out of this mold is necessary if we're to move in a direction of improving our overall health and well-being – putting our trust in what have now become "out of the box" remedies, but which are in fact just good old simple natural solutions that don't make money for big pharma. Keep in mind that in many instances, with natural remedies, the proof is in

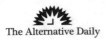

the use. Big research dollars for natural remedies just don't exist, and this is one of the reasons why you don't see a boatload of research on ACV. What does exist, however, makes a very strong case for its effectiveness.

We hope that you gain as much pleasure and insight into the bounties that nature has to offer by reading this book as we did researching and writing it.

What Do We Know About Raw, Organic Apple Cider Vinegar?

Raw, organic ACV is made from sweet, fall varieties of organic apples. These apples undergo a double fermentation process, which produces enzymes and creates many of the vinegar's health-promoting characteristics. As sugar in the apples is broken down, the first ferment yields what we know as "hard" cider, or alcoholic cider. The second fermentation brings forth ACV.

Organic ACV is unpasteurized and contains what is known as mother of vinegar, which makes the vinegar appear somewhat cloudy. Also known as Mycoderma aceti, Mother of vinegar is created when acetic acid bacteria and a type of cellulose develop during the fermentation process. Mother of vinegar is harmless, contains health-promoting characteristics such as living nutrients and friendly

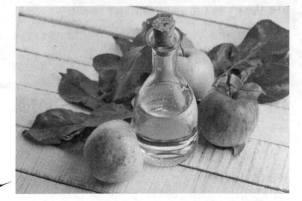

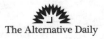
The Alternative Daily

bacteria, and lets you know that the vinegar is unpasteurized. Most vinegar manufacturers nowadays pasteurize the vinegar before it hits the shelves, to get rid

of the mother of vinegar, and in turn, a lot of the nutrients that the vinegar offers.

When choosing an ACV, make sure to select one that is raw, organic and unpasteurized, as the pasteurization process can destroy many of the health benefits. Organic, unpasteurized ACV has a cobweb-looking solid floating inside; this is known as mother of vinegar, and is a natural cellulose produced by the vinegar bacteria.

Beneficial Properties

Some of the beneficial properties contained within mother of vinegar include:

- **Potassium:** essential for healthy metabolism, as well as water and chemical balance in the body
- **Iron:** important for blood health
- **Magnesium:** vital to heart health
- **Enzymes:** boost chemical reactions in the body
- **Malic acid:** protects vinegar from viruses, bacteria and fungus
- **Acetic acid:** slows the digestion of starch and inhibits bacterial growth
- **Calcium:** builds strong bones and teeth
- **Pectin:** helps regulate blood pressure and cholesterol
- **Ash:** maintains a healthy alkaline state in the body

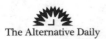

Other Minerals, Trace Elements and Vitamins

- Chlorine
- Copper
- Fluorine
- Phosphorous
- Pro-vitamin beta-carotene
- Silicon
- Sodium
- Vitamin A
- Vitamin B1
- Vitamin B2
- Vitamin B6
- Vitamin C
- Vitamin E
- Vitamin P

More Powerhouse Properties

Alkalinity: A big reason why ACV is so effective for so many conditions is because it makes the body alkaline, as opposed to acidic. The more acidic your body is, the better the environment for sickness and disease to take hold (see pH Balance #26). Even though ACV is acidic, it has an alkalinizing impact on the body during digestion, unlike other vinegars.

The 3 A's: ACV contains potent antifungal, antibacterial and antiviral properties, which help to make it so effective for so many conditions.

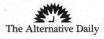
The Alternative Daily

Detoxifier: Toxins often accumulate in our bodies, and the malic acid in ACV helps to eliminate these dangerous compounds. By doing so, ACV supports healthy kidney, bladder and liver function.

A Word About Potassium Deficiency

We all know that the advice given for high blood pressure is to cut down on sodium. But very rarely are we told about how important increasing potassium intake really is.

Potassium is a mineral – an electrolyte – that balances the acidity and alkalinity in body fluids and also helps to control blood pressure.

With the emergence of industrialized agricultural practices, the amount of potassium that humans consume has decreased significantly. At one time, humans ate a diet high in potassium and low in sodium, versus a diet that is now high in sodium and low in potassium.

With an increase in processed foods and the decreased consumption of fruits and vegetables, many people suffer from a lack of potassium. Interestingly enough, in developing countries, where diets are not processed, high blood pressure is a rare occurrence.

Why is Potassium so Important?

Potassium controls the electrical activity of the heart, builds protein and helps to break down carbohydrates. Recent research indicates that a diet rich in potassium provides protection from heart disease, stroke, hypertension, kidney disease and even osteoporosis. In an epidemiological study of over 80,000 women, potassium was found to lower the risk of diabetes, as well.

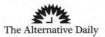

A study performed at Harvard Medical School was published in the journal Hypertension by St. George's Medical School of London. This study compared the effectiveness of dietary potassium and potassium supplements in reducing blood pressure. According to the study, there were no differences between the two; dietary potassium was as effective as the supplements in reducing blood pressure.

How Much Potassium is Enough?

While U.S. governmental guidelines recommend that we get 4,700 mg of potassium per day, author and medical expert Dr. Steven G. Pratt suggests that we need more like 8,000 mg. However, if you suffer from kidney disease you will want to speak with your physician about possibly avoiding both sodium and potassium.

How Do I Know if My Potassium is Low?

The body gives us warning signs when our potassium levels drop dangerously low. This condition is known as hypokalemia. It is paramount to stay in tune with these warning signs and understand what they may mean. Some signs to watch for are:

- Weakness
- Low energy
- Irregular heartbeat
- Muscle cramps
- Dizziness
- Morning headaches

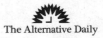
The Alternative Daily

- Dull and faded hair
- Itchy eyes
- Mental fatigue
- Depression
- Anxiety
- Cold hands and feet

Foods that Offer Potassium

Here are some great sources of potassium to consider including in your diet. If you consume a diet of highly refined foods and rarely eat fruits and vegetables, eating some of these nutrient-dense foods can improve your overall health and well-being.

- **Sweet Potato** – 1 cup cooked – 950 mg potassium
- **Butternut squash** – 1 cup cooked – 582 mg potassium
- **Figs** – 4 large – 541 mg potassium
- **Cantaloupe** – 1 cup – 494 mg potassium
- **Lentils** – ½ cup cooked – 475 mg potassium
- **Avocado** – ½ medium – 439 mg potassium
- **Bananas** – 1 medium – 422 mg potassium
- **Spinach** – 2 cups raw – 334 mg potassium
- **Apple** - 1 large – 290 mg potassium
- **Blackberries** – 1 cup – 282 mg potassium
- **Strawberries** – 1 cup – 252 mg potassium
- **Almonds** – 1 ounce raw – 198 mg potassium

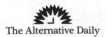

ACV contains a high amount of potassium, and using it daily can help replenish your potassium supply - leaving you feeling refreshed and vibrant.

A Word of Caution

Keep in mind that ACV is highly acidic, so it is always best to dilute it. Straight apple cider vinegar may damage tooth enamel or burn mouth and throat tissue.

ACV may interact with diuretics and other medicines, so be sure to check with a healthcare provider before using.

Apple cider vinegar can be found in pill form, but it is best to consume it fresh and in juice form because processing changes its healing properties

Apple Cider Vinegar for Exceptional Health

"A wise man ought to realize that health is his most valuable possession."~Hippocrates

The benefits of living a healthy lifestyle are practically endless. By eating a balanced, nutritious diet, exercising regularly, practicing stress reduction techniques and getting enough rest you will do much to improve your quality of life, and possibly even increase its duration.

The natural world is full of the raw materials that we need to be healthy. Adding ACV to an already healthy and clean lifestyle is just one way that you can utilize a simple, natural provision that costs so little for what it has to offer.

Here are 81 of our top ways that you can incorporate the healing and cleansing properties of well-fermented organic apples into your life.

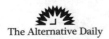

#1 Weight Loss/Fat Breakdown

It is a well-known fact that obesity is seriously hazardous to one's health. The increased risk of type 2 diabetes, cardiovascular disease and stroke that obese individuals face has been heavily researched, and the number of obese children and adults is still on the rise.

While there is no replacement for a healthy diet and exercise to manage weight, ACV does seem to show some potential for managing hunger and weight control.

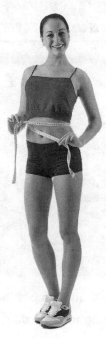

Vinegars of all kinds have been used for a very long time as a weight loss aid because they help make you feel full. A study conducted with 12 people found that those who ate a piece of bread with ACV felt fuller than those who ate the bread alone.

In another study, overweight Japanese participants were grouped based on body weight, body mass index (BMI) and waist size. Members of each group drank 30 ml, 15 ml or 0 ml of this vinegar per day for 12 weeks. The people who drank 30 ml and 15 ml had lower BMI, waist circumference and visceral fat than those in the control group, who did not drink apple cider vinegar.

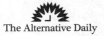
The Alternative Daily

Amino acids found in proteins must be broken down so that they can fuel a number of important processes in the body. ACV helps the body break down proteins - some of which are integral in the creation of growth hormone. Growth hormone is vital to weight loss in that it helps to break down fat found in cells.

Application

Mix 2 tablespoons of ACV with filtered water, and drink about 10 minutes before each meal for best impact.

#2 Hangover Helper

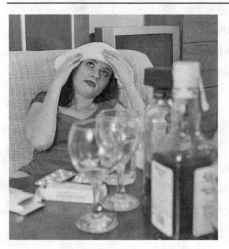

Consuming alcohol leaves toxins in our bodies, which contribute to that nasty hangover feeling. ACV helps to balance pH levels while replenishing minerals including potassium, calcium, iron, sodium and magnesium. What does this mean for you? It means that you will recover much quicker. Mix 2 tablespoons of ACV into 8 ounces of filtered water and drink - repeat this 2 more times throughout the day.

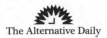

#3 Cancer

If we just implemented a few simple, healthy strategies into our daily lives, we could dramatically reduce the number of cancer deaths in this country, according to the American Cancer Society's annual report, *Cancer Prevention and Early Detection Facts and Figures.*

An estimated 585,720 people will die from cancer in 2014, according to the report. Nearly a third of these deaths will be due to tobacco use alone. An additional third of cancer deaths will be caused by obesity and being overweight, lack of physical activity and poor diet, the organization says.

Apple cider vinegar may kill cancer cells or retard their growth. According to one study, consuming organic apple cider vinegar decreased the risk of esophageal cancer. In clinical trials, pectin, contained in apple cider vinegar, was shown to slow the growth of cancerous cells within the prostate. Apple cider vinegar cleanses the colon, which also supports a healthy prostate.

According to Charlotte Gerson of the Gerson Institute, ACV promotes alkalinity, and cancer can't survive in an alkaline environment. The Gerson Therapy fights against cancer by bringing the body into an alkaline state.

Application

Take 2 tablespoons of ACV in filtered water 3 times a day before meals. If you need it a bit sweeter, add some raw honey or stevia.

#4 Nosebleeds

If you are injured or prone to nosebleeds, soak a cotton ball in ACV and lightly pack your nostril. Lean forward for 10 minutes, pressing nostrils together. ACV contains properties that help constrict blood vessels and slow bleeding.

#5 External Itching ×××

Itching can be downright annoying, and applying many over-the-counter creams can only make matters worse. Because ACV has antibiotic properties, it can help reduce inflammation and relieve the source of your itch. Mix ¼ cup ACV with 1 cup water and apply to the itchy area with a clean cotton ball. Repeat as necessary.

APPLE FACT: It takes the energy of 50 leaves to produce 1 apple.

#6 Sore Throat ×××

The antibacterial properties of ACV can help to neutralize infections that cause sore throats while reducing inflammation. Mix ¼ cup ACV with ¼ cup filtered water and gargle with this solution for at least 30 seconds, then rinse with water.

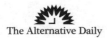

#7 Athletes Foot

Athlete's food is a fungal infection that can cause burning, itching and inflammation. ACV has antifungal properties that can kill the fungus and keep it from returning. Put 2 ounces of ACV in a spray bottle and spray on dry feet. Pat dry after application and moisturize with olive or coconut oil. You can also soak your feet in a foot bath with 2 tablespoons of Himalayan salt crystals, ½ cup of ACV and warm water.

TRY IT: Sprinkle your toes with some organic cornstarch before putting on your socks. The cornstarch will absorb excess moisture.

#8 Strengthen Bones

ACV contains magnesium, manganese, silicon and calcium, which have all been found to be effective against osteoporosis. Mix 2 tablespoons ACV with 1 tablespoon raw honey and 8 ounces of water. Drink 3 times daily, preferably before meals.

#9 Diarrhea

Although many things can cause diarrhea and it is sometimes just a way that the body rids itself of dangerous compounds, it should not be ignored. The pectin in ACV helps to form bulk in the stool, which works against diarrhea and also works to eliminate the bacteria that cause it. In the intestines, gut flora help to turn pectin into a soothing coating that protects the irritated colon. Mix 2 tablespoons of ACV with 1 tablespoon of raw honey and 8 ounces of water, and sip the mixture throughout the day.

#*10* Diabetes

Most of the scientific data collected on ACV has been done with regards to its impact on blood sugar. Type 2 diabetes is a lifelong chronic condition with serious negative effects on your entire body. It can cause everything from kidney failure and blindness to heart disease and stroke, nerve damage and even the loss of fingers, toes or entire limbs. Obesity is thought to be the main cause of type 2 diabetes in those who are genetically predisposed.

DID YOU KNOW: It's been estimated that as many as 79 million people in the US have been diagnosed with pre-diabetes, which means they are at high risk of developing type 2 diabetes, and also have a significant risk of developing heart disease.

Unless those diagnosed with pre-diabetes adopt a healthier lifestyle that includes regular exercise and weight loss, they will likely develop the disease within a decade, if not much sooner.

One study, conducted at Arizona State University by Doctors Carol S. Johnston and Andrea M. White, PhD, surveyed 11 people afflicted with type 2 diabetes. The researchers found that taking two tablespoons of apple cider vinegar right before bed lowered the blood sugar levels of these individuals by four to six percent by morning.

Another study led by Dr. Johnston gave subjects, some with insulin resistance and some without, 20 grams of apple cider vinegar and 40 grams

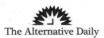

of water. Results showed that the after-meal blood sugar levels of the subjects with insulin resistance lowered by 34 percent when they drank the apple cider vinegar.

Dr. Johnston says, "scientific studies over the past 10 years show benefits from vinegar consumption. It's inexpensive and can be easily incorporated into the diet. Used in combination with diet and exercise, it can help many people with type 2 diabetes."

At Tokyo University in Tokyo, Japan, it was discovered that the acetic acid found in vinegars inhibits the activity of carbohydrate-digesting enzymes, including sucrase, maltase, lactase and amylase. This inhibition results in select sugars and starches passing through the digestive system without being digested, having less impact on blood sugar levels.

Application

Drink 2 tablespoons of ACV in distilled water 3 times a day before meals to manage blood sugar.

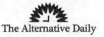

#11 Carpal Tunnel Syndrome

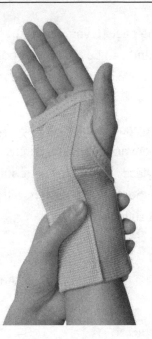

Carpal tunnel syndrome occurs when the nerve which runs from the forearm to the palm of the hand is pressed or squeezed at the wrist. Many people who work long days with their hands or in a repetitive fashion suffer from this condition. Because ACV contains anti-inflammatory properties, it has been used as an effective remedy for carpal tunnel. If you are bothered by the pain of carpal tunnel syndrome, mix 1 tablespoon of ACV with 8 ounces of water and drink 3 times a day on an empty stomach.

#12 Blood Pressure

Elevated blood pressure is a major cause of heart disease and stroke. Every year, over half a million people die from heart disease, and the numbers are on the rise. High blood pressure also causes kidney disease, dementia and some eye problems.

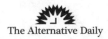

The cause of high blood pressure is often misunderstood. Organs need oxygen, which is carried through the body by the blood, in order to survive. As the heart beats, it creates pressure that forces the blood through blood vessels and capillaries. This pressure - known as blood pressure - is the result of two forces. The first force occurs when blood pumps out of the heart (systolic) and into the arteries and the second force results as the heart rests between the heart beats (diastolic). Major risk factors for high blood pressure include abdominal obesity, smoking and stress.

What high blood pressure does

Arteries that are healthy are comprised of muscles and semi-flexible tissue that stretches out when the heart pumps blood. The more forcefully the blood pumps, the more the arteries stretch to allow the blood through. If the force of the blood is too high for an extended period of time, the artery walls stretch too much, creating vascular weakness which makes them prone to rupture. It also causes vascular scarring, which can catch debris such as cholesterol, blood cells and plaque. This can lead to an increased risk of blood clots, heart attack and stroke.

Research suggests that apple cider vinegar may lower blood pressure and reduce the risk of heart disease. Potassium is known as a "detergent for the arteries," because it will flush out and cleanse arterial walls and drag excess sodium from the body. ACV will also help to keep the body alkaline (especially if combined with baking soda), which helps to

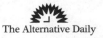
The Alternative Daily

further reduce your blood pressure. In addition, this vinegar also contains magnesium, which helps to relax blood vessel walls, resulting in a lowering of blood pressure.

Application

Dilute 1 tablespoon of ACV in 8 ounces of filtered water. Drink this 3 times a day.

DID YOU KNOW: 30 minutes of brisk walking daily can lower your blood pressure.

"Our bodies are our gardens – our wills are our gardeners."
~William Shakespeare

#13 Leg Cramps

If you have leg cramps, you may be running low on potassium. Eating potassium rich foods such as bananas and drinking ACV daily can help to restore your potassium levels. Mix 2 tablespoons of ACV with 8 ounces of warm water and drink 3 times a day to relieve cramps. You can add some raw honey or stevia to sweeten the drink.

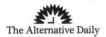

#14 Edema

Mix 1 ounce ACV with 1 ounce distilled water. Soak cotton pads in the mixture and apply to the affected areas for 5 minutes. Repeat 3 times a day. ACV will help alleviate the pain caused by edema by reducing swelling.

TRY IT: If you suffer from edema, reduce or eliminate processed sugar and refined salt from your diet. Consume lots of fresh fruits and vegetables and plenty of pure water.

#15 Hay Fever

Mix 2 teaspoons of ACV with 2 teaspoons of local, raw honey in a glass of warm water. Drink this 3 times a day during hay fever season. ACV works as a natural antihistamine and has been touted by many as an all-season remedy for hay fever.

#16 Bed Wetting

Mix 2 drops of ACV in 6 ounces of water and drink at least one hour before bed. ACV helps to reduce acid levels in the stomach, which often contribute to excessive bed wetting.

#*17* Heartburn

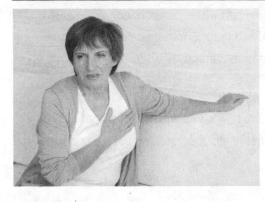

Fact: 90 percent of the time, heartburn is caused by too little stomach acid, not too much.

Not having enough stomach acid (hypochlorhydria) can significantly impact digestive health. A normal stomach that makes enough acid has a pH between 1 and 3. In a stomach that does not make enough acid, the pH is between 4 and 7. If you don't have enough hydrochloric acid, your stomach cannot initiate the production of pepsin, which is necessary to break down proteins properly.

Proteins break down into amino acids and peptides. If you suffer from insomnia, depression or brain fog, or are having a hard time building muscle, it may be caused by a lack of amino acids. Lacking certain amino acids can lead to neurotransmitter problems. If you want to put on muscle, you need proteins to break down properly.

If the chyme coming out of the stomach is not acidic enough, the liver and gallbladder do not function properly, which means the bile cannot break down fats, and the pancreas malfunctions. This leads to deficiencies in fatty acids such as omega-6, and problems with the fat-soluble vitamins A, D, E, and K.

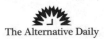

Sufficient stomach acid also protects you from dangerous bacteria and parasites that are found on and in food. When stomach acid is at the normal pH, most parasites and bacteria can't survive for more than 15 minutes. However, when you have too little stomach acid and your pH is high, parasites and bacteria pass through the stomach and set up shop in your body, which can lead to heartburn.

Bacteria that come in through food and drink feed off of carbohydrates. Without enough stomach acid, you also do not have enough amylase and other enzymes needed to break down carbohydrates.

The bacteria, now present in your stomach, feed happily on all of the unbroken pieces of carbohydrates. As this happens, you become bloated and gassy. The gas pushes back through the stomach, opens the LES valve and allows the acid to enter the esophagus, causing heartburn.

Rather than reach for over-the-counter antacids, which only mask problems with acid reflux and heartburn, try to give your stomach the acid that it needs to balance. ACV helps to break food down by mimicking the stomach environment.

Application

Take a tablespoon of ACV with a glass of water, and the burning should subside in a few minutes. If the burning becomes worse, see your physician, as this could be a sign that you have an ulcer.

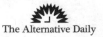

#18 Chronic Fatigue

Chronic fatigue syndrome (CFS) is known to devastate lives; although the exact number affected is unknown, it is estimated that there are at least 3 million people in the US with CFS. There have been a variety of theories as to what causes it, including a weak immune system, infections, and even some "experts" stating that it is "all in your head."

Symptoms of chronic fatigue can be quite debilitating, and include memory loss, sore throat, fever, joint and muscle pain, headaches, confusion, lack of concentration and sore lymph nodes.

It is thought that one of the main causes of chronic fatigue is a lack of good, sound sleep. Even though you may go to bed early, you may still not sleep well and wake up feeling exhausted and sore. When potassium levels in the body fall low, muscles can build up lactic acid, and this can be very painful.

The potassium in apple cider vinegar helps to break down the lactic acid, thereby reducing muscle stiffness and soreness.

Application:

Mix 3 tablespoons of apple cider vinegar with 1 cup of local, pure honey, and take 2 tablespoons as needed.

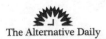

19 Workout Endurance

Do you often feel fatigued halfway through your workout? While you are working out, lactic acid collects in your muscles and contributes to a heavy and fatigued feeling. ACV helps to push the toxins out of your body and balances pH. For an extra boost to get you through a tough routine, mix 1 tablespoon of ACV in 8 ounces of distilled water and drink during your workout. Follow this with 8 ounces of pure, filtered water.

#*20* Headaches

There is nothing quite so distracting as a pounding headache. Headaches can range from mild to severe, even temporarily debilitating. There are many different types of headaches, caused by any number of things including dehydration, allergies, poor diet, sinus problems, lack of sleep, stress and hormones.

Headaches can also occur from a toxic build-up inside of the body. A headache is a warning sign that something is amiss, whether it be in the gallbladder, liver, kidney, bowel or any of the body's other organs.

Because headaches can be so painful, sufferers often desire imme-diate relief and resort to over-the-counter or even prescription medica-tion. There are several problems with this, including the fact that some prescription painkillers can become addictive and cause other long term health problems.

In addition, people who depend on popular headache medicines, such as Advil or Tylenol, may experience what is known as rebound headaches. Rebound headaches occur when the brain becomes overstimulated.

The malic acid in ACV works to return the body to a balanced pH by supporting healthy kidney function. In many cases, this can help to reduce the frequency of headaches.

Application

Fill a large glass mixing bowl with boiling hot water and add one cup of ACV. Place your head under a towel so that you face is right over the bowl. Take deep breaths in and out - keep your breathing steady - for about 10 minutes or until the water cools. Be careful not to get your face too close to the steam.

You can also dip an organic cotton face towel in the warm ACV and water and wring it out (being careful not to burn your hands). Place the cloth on the back of your neck and lie down for about 15 minutes until you feel relaxed. This is especially effective for migraines.

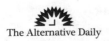

"To ensure good health: eat lightly, breathe deeply, live moderately, cultivate cheerfulness, and maintain an interest in life." ~William Londen

#21 Cholesterol

Today, over 40 million people around the world are prescribed statins to lower cholesterol and to prevent cardiovascular disease. However, more and more research is showing that statins may do much more harm than good. A new study has linked statin use with a higher risk of developing diabetes.

One of the most frightening facts about statins is that in 75 percent of cases, they are prescribed to healthy individuals for preventative purposes, as a 'primary prevention' measure against heart disease. However, overwhelming research shows that using statins for primary prevention does nothing to increase life expectancy.

With more people seeking out alternatives to pharmaceuticals, the use of ACV is starting to gain some traction. The impact that ACV has on regulating cholesterol has been studied and has yielded favorable results.

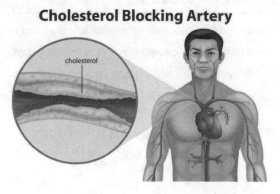

Cholesterol Blocking Artery

cholesterol

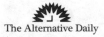
The Alternative Daily

The British Journal of Nutrition published a study done on rats that investigated ACV and cholesterol. Scientists were able to see that the acetic acid in ACV lowered bad cholesterol.

In Japan, a manufacturer of condiments, Mizkan, did some independent research and found that 15 milliliters of ACV daily reduces blood cholesterol in humans.

Application

Take 1 tablespoon of ACV mixed in 8 ounces of water daily to help regulate blood cholesterol.

#22 Chicken Pox

Relieve itching by mixing 1 cup of ACV in 5 cups of filtered water. Wash the affected areas with a clean cloth dipped in the mixture. This will help reduce swelling and will also help keep the infection from spreading.

#23 Back Pain

Because ACV has anti-inflammatory and antioxidant properties, it can relieve back pain caused by injury. Soak a cotton pad in 2 ounces of ACV and apply it to the sore area. To relieve pain associated with lactic acid buildup, drink 2 tablespoons of ACV mixed in 8 ounces of filtered water.

APPLE FACT: Apples are members of the rose family.

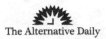

#24 Epilepsy

To calm the nervous system and improve digestion (both of which help reduce symptoms of epilepsy), mix 1 tablespoon of ACV with 8 ounces of filtered water and drink on an empty stomach 3 times a day.

#25 Jock Itch

Relieve pain associated with jock itch by mixing 1 teaspoon of ACV in 1 cup of water. Apply to the affected area with a clean cotton pad; leave it on for 10 minutes and rinse the area with water. Repeat this 3 times daily and before bed.

#26 pH Balance

Over-acidity, which is highly common today, is a dangerous condition that contributes to a host of serious health conditions. An acidic internal environment is the perfect place for disease to thrive. This is opposed to a pH balanced environment, in which normal body function resists disease. In a healthy body, there are alkaline reserves, which are used in times of emergency to balance internal pH. When too many acids enter the body, the reserves become depleted, leaving the body weak and vulnerable. Health experts warn that a pH balanced diet is necessary to maintaining health.

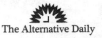

Acidosis is extremely common in our society, mostly due to the American diet and lifestyle. Although eggs, dairy and meats are acidic, the main problem is with processed foods. These include white flour, sugar, coffee and soda, which create an acidic environment.

Drugs are also acid-forming, as are artificial sweeteners such as Equal and NutraSweet. One of the first things that needs to be done to regulate pH levels inside the body is to stop eating processed foods and start eating a clean diet. In addition, stress, smoking and lack of exercise all contribute to acidity.

FACT: Many people are too acidic. When this condition prevails, the body steals minerals such as sodium, potassium and calcium from bones and organs to neutralize the acid and escort it out of the body. This puts tremendous strain on the body and, unfortunately, can go unnoticed for years.

Even mild acidosis can cause such health problems as fatigue, depression, infections, obesity, dry skin, ulcers, diabetes, immune deficiency, hormone issues, premature aging, weak bones, yeast, slow digestion, bladder conditions, kidney problems, cardiovascular damage and joint pain due to lactic acid buildup.

In addition to eating an alkaline diet that emphasizes fresh fruits and vegetables, ACV can help restore internal pH balance. Because it is alkaline in nature, it is a natural way to help the body regain the proper pH level: between 7.35 and 7.45.

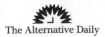

Application

To balance pH, mix 2 tablespoons of ACV in 8 ounces of filtered water and drink 3 times a day before meals. Add one teaspoon of raw honey or stevia to sweeten. This mixture can be drunk warm or cold.

"A man too busy to take care of his health is like a mechanic too busy to take care of his tools." ~ Spanish Proverb

#27 Constipation

Constipation is an annoying and often painful condition suffered by millions of Americans. If you have less than three stools per week, you are constipated. If you have less than one stool per week, you are severely constipated.

The cause of constipation can be traced back to any number of things, including poor diet, medication, poor bowel habits, dehydration, hormonal disorders and laxative abuse. For many people, the discomfort of constipation becomes so great that they reach for over-the-counter medications for relief. Unfortunately, many of these medications only mask the symptoms and can make the problem worse.

Before doing anything else, it is imperative to have a look at your diet. People who consume too few fats in their diet tend to have a problem using the bathroom more frequently than those who get enough fat. Healthy fats, such as those found in olive oil, nuts, coconut oil, avocados, olives, fatty fresh-caught fish and flaxseed oil, are great additions to your diet.

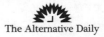

These fats not only help keep the digestive system lubricated, they also fight off obesity, improve cognitive function and increase energy. Aim for a little fat with each meal, and stay clear of the fats in processed foods – they will only exacerbate problems in the digestive system.

The benefit of fiber in the diet should never be underplayed. Both insoluble and soluble fiber are necessary for healthy elimination. Insoluble fiber passes through the body virtually unchanged. It provides bulk for stools and makes them easier to pass by keeping their texture smooth.

Foods that have a high amount of insoluble fiber include fruits, vegetables and whole grains. Soluble fiber is found in foods such as oatmeal, legumes, fruits and green vegetables. This fiber dissolves in water and makes a gel-type substance in the intestines. Soluble fiber slows digestion and allows the body to absorb as many nutrients as possible from food.

In addition to changing your diet, a natural laxative made with ACV can help to keep your bowel function regular.

Application

Mix 1 tablespoon raw honey with 2 tablespoons ACV and 1 cup of water. Drink on an empty stomach before breakfast and 30 minutes before going to bed.

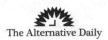

BEWARE OF THE GHOST POOP

There are many things in life worth hanging onto, but a bowel movement is not one of these things. If you suppress the urge to use the bathroom repeatedly, ignoring the signs, you become less sensitive to the movement of your bowels. The urge to go move your bowels goes away, which is known as a "Ghost Poop." This leads to constipation. It is essential to use the bathroom when you need to in order to avoid an uncomfortable and unhealthy back-up.

#28 Candida

You have probably heard the word candida, but may not be exactly sure what it is. Candida is a fungus, which is actually a form of yeast. Everyone has a small amount of yeast living in their mouth and intestines. It serves an important role when it comes to digestion and nutrient absorption, but when it overpopulates, it actually breaks down the walls of the intestines and seeps into the bloodstream, where it releases toxins. This leakage can cause a number of health conditions, ranging from digestive disturbances to depression.

We all have a certain amount of healthy gut bacteria, which works to keep yeast levels healthy. However, many things can lead to candida getting out of control and overpowering the healthy bacteria. The good news is, we have control over most, if not all, of the factors contributing to this, which include:

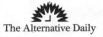
The Alternative Daily

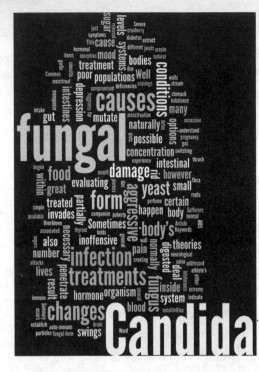

Eating a diet loaded with refined sugar and carbohydrates – A diet rich in sugar or anything that converts to sugar, such as processed foods made with refined grains and alcohol, all encourage yeast growth. The sugar creates a perfect environment for the yeast to thrive, and they quickly multiply.

Taking oral contraceptives – Taking a birth control pill causes an upset in hormones, which disrupts the good bacteria in the gut.

Living a very high stress life – When you are stressed, your body releases cortisol, a hormone that depresses your immune system and increases blood sugar. The yeast feeds on the increased sugar, the immune system is too weak to stop it and growth gets out of hand. In addition, if you remain stressed for a long period of time, your adrenal glands become ineffective and your immune system can be further compromised.

Antibiotics - While antibiotics effectively kill the harmful bacteria that make you sick, they also kill the friendly bacteria in your digestive system. This leaves you defenseless to fungus and yeast, which can quickly take over your gut.

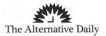

Do I have a yeast problem?

Many people have a variety of the symptoms of candida overgrowth, but fail to connect the dots and put them all together. Here are just a few of the warning signs to watch out for:

- Fungal infections on skin or nails, such as athlete's foot or toenail fungus
- Fatigue or fibromyalgia
- Constipation, bloating or diarrhea
- Bad breath
- Dry mouth
- Joint pain
- Numbness
- Hair loss
- Headaches
- PMS
- Heartburn
- Burning eyes
- Lack of impulse control
- Hyperactivity
- Poor concentration, brain fog, lack of focus, ADD or ADHD
- Autoimmune diseases such as rheumatoid arthritis, lupus, ulcerative colitis or multiple sclerosis

- Mood swings, anxiety or depression
- Strong cravings for sugar or refined carbohydrates
- Skin conditions such as eczema, psoriasis, rashes or hives
- Seasonal allergies or itchy ears
- Urinary tract infections, vaginal or rectal itching

Foods that encourage yeast

The following foods can create yeast overgrowth, or make an already existing yeast problem much worse:

- Breads
- Pizza
- Fast food
- Dairy
- Soda
- Juice
- Alcohol
- Fruit

TRY IT: Spit Test for Yeast

Yeah, we know, it sounds a little gross, but a spit test offers a really good analysis of what is going on inside your body, and may give you a sign that yeast is the problem. The best time to take this test is as soon as you wake up in the morning, before you even get out of bed.

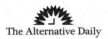

Here is how you do it:

1. Gather as much spit as possible from inside your mouth.

2. Spit into a clear glass filled with room temperature filtered water.

3. Watch carefully.

4. The saliva will float at first - watch to see if there are thin projections extending downward into the water after 15 minutes or so. They may look like hairs or strings. If this happens, you may have a candida overgrowth problem.

5. If your saliva is very cloudy and sinks to the bottom within a few minutes, or parts of the saliva slowly sink, yeast overgrowth is a possibility. The particles are yeast colonies which band together.

6. If your spit is still floating after about an hour, it is likely that your yeast is under control.

I think I have yeast, what now?

According to the National Candida Center, if you have symptoms and your spit test is positive for yeast, it is a pretty good indication that you have a candida overgrowth problem. The first step in addressing the problem is to adjust your diet.

Eliminate all processed foods and sugars, and begin eating only wholesome foods, organic if possible. Adding ACV to your diet will also help eliminate toxins and kill yeast overgrowth.

A 2011 study published in the *Thi-Qar Medical Journal* found that the primary component of ACV that is responsible for its antifungal action is acetic acid. The same study also noted that ACV was more effective than Fluconazole, a standard antifungal drug.

Application

When used in conjunction with an anti-candida diet, ACV can help kill and control candida overgrowth.

Warm Drink:

Mix 2 tablespoons of ACV with 1 cup of warm water. Add 1 teaspoon of blackstrap molasses. Drink this mixture slowly before meals. Because a fair amount of yeast and bacteria will die off in your stomach, you may feel dizzy or nauseous for a time; this is normal. To ease these symptoms, take a hot bath with 2 cups of Epsom salts.

ACV Bath:

For vaginal yeast, fill a bath with warm water (just enough to cover your belly) and add 2 cups of ACV. Bathe in the solution with your knees pulled up for 15 minutes per day to reduce the symptoms of vaginal yeast infections.

#29 Nail Fungus

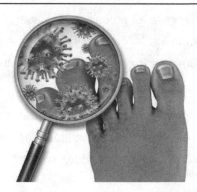

Nail fungus is unsightly and can be painful. This fungus begins as a white spot and eventually becomes a yellow spot under the tip of your finger or toenail. The fungus will spread and go deeper into your nail, causing it to discolor and thicken

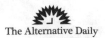

with crumbling edges. ACV can be used to help with nail fungus in two ways; you can drink 2 tablespoons of ACV mixed in 8 ounces of water 3 times daily to help balance pH, and also massage a mixture of 2 tablespoons ACV and 1 tablespoon water into your nail 3 times a day.

#30 Varicose Veins

Varicose veins and hemorrhoids are two examples of swollen veins. This condition may result from a number of things, including excess weight, heavy lifting, birth control, heredity, occupations that involve standing for long periods of time or hormonal changes. No matter what the cause, swollen veins are both unsightly and uncomfortable. Conventional treatments for this condition include pharmaceuticals or surgery, however, a number of natural therapies including ACV may bring great relief. Additional relief may come from elevating your feet as much as possible, wearing comfortable and supportive shoes and consuming plenty of pure water daily.

Application

Soak a cotton wrap in ACV and wring it out. Wrap your legs and elevate them for about 20 minutes daily. Repeat as often as necessary to help reduce swelling and pain. This is especially effective if you have been on your feet for a long period of time.

#31 Erectile Dysfunction

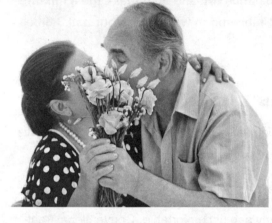

Older guys with expanding waistlines (40 inches plus) are at risk for more than just another pair of Sans-a-Belt pants. They're chancing diabetes, heart disease, cancer and mental dysfunction, along with some below-the-belt problems. To spice up your love life, start moving and embracing a healthy diet. In addition to this, try mixing 1 tablespoon of ACV into 8 ounces of distilled water and drinking the mixture 3 times a day. ACV is known as a natural blood thinner and helps to improve circulation.

#32 Corns, Calluses and Warts

Corns usually occur when shoes don't fit right. If the are too tight the toes press against each other, and if they are too loose there can be friction on the feet. Corns are generally small, yellow or gray in color and quite painful because they can press on nerve endings. Calluses may occur on any part of the body, but are usually found on joints and weight-bearing

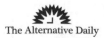

areas such as the palms, or the sides and soles of feet. Generally, calluses are not painful, just unsightly. Warts are caused by a viral infection and can be painful if left untreated. Unlike calluses or corns, warts are contagious.

The conventional manner of removal for corns, calluses and warts involves the use of salicylic acid, however ACV is also an effective and very safe method for removal.

Application

Calluses: Fill a wash tub with warm water and add ⅓ cup of ACV. Soak the affected area for about 20 minutes. Dry with a towel and use a pumice stone to gently brush the area. After this, pour a little full-strength ACV on a piece of gauze and cover the affected area overnight. In the morning, replace the gauze with a new one and continue the treatment until the calluses dissolve. Be sure to also get a good pair of shoes that fit, and walk barefoot on the grass or sand when you can.

Corns: Mix 1 ounce of ACV with 1 ounce of tea tree oil and soak a cotton ball in the mixture. Apply to the corn and allow it to set for 5 minutes. Dry by patting with a soft cloth and repeat the procedure again. Follow this method until you see the corn start to peel up. At this time, rub lightly with a pumice stone to smooth the area.

Warts: For common warts, follow the calluses procedure, only be very careful not to rub the warts as this could cause them to spread. For daytime treatment use a castor-oil soaked gauze bandage. Continue until the wart is gone.

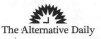
The Alternative Daily

#33 Head Lice

Although lice are not dangerous and don't spread infection, they are an annoying and very common childhood problem that can spread rapidly through a school classroom. Eggs from head lice are hard to remove because the female lice lay them on strands of hair and actually cement them in place with a substance that is sticky like glue. Commercial lice products contain chemicals, and are often not that effective in lice removal. Instead of spending a great deal of money on products from your drugstore, try ACV therapy instead. Mix 1 cup of ACV in 8 ounces of mineral oil. Coat the hair and scalp with the mixture and cover with shower cap. Leave the cap on overnight. Wash the hair in the morning as usual. Be sure to wash all bedding, clothing and other infected materials and surfaces well.

#34 Ear Infections

There are many reasons why ear infections occur, ranging from a foreign object lodged in the ear to wax buildup or bacteria. Whatever the cause, an ear infection is a painful condition that can leave both children and adults irritable and uncomfortable.

Many times, ear infections are treated with antibiotics. However, antibiotics are not always effective, have some disturbing side effects and are often over-prescribed, which leads to antibiotic resistance. According to the CDC, antibiotic resistance is a leading world health problem. Doctors

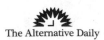

first began to notice resistance problems almost a decade ago when kids with middle-ear infections stopped responding to the drugs they were being given.

Dr. Robert O. Young and Shelley Redford Young, authors of the book *The pH Miracle*, note that ACV creates an environment in the ear where viruses cannot survive, and helps to alleviate the pain associated with an infection.

ACV is also noted to be effective against swimmer's ear, a condition that results from swimming and showering.

Application:

Make ACV eardrops by gently warming some ACV on the stove on low heat. Test the vinegar on your wrist to find the right temperature - be careful not to overheat. Using a dropper, place a few drops into one ear and cover the ear opening with a cotton ball. It is best to have the patient lying down with the ear facing up to allow the solution to penetrate.

#35 Sinus Congestion

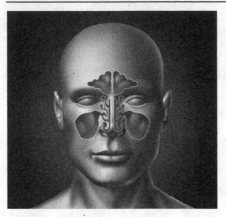

Because ACV breaks up mucus in the body, it can bring quite a bit of relief to those suffering with chronic sinusitis. Drink 1 cup of water mixed with 2 tablespoons of ACV before meals. You can also fill a steam vaporizer with 1 cup of ACV and hot water and inhale the steam.

"He who cures a disease may be the skillfullest, but he that prevents it is the safest physician."
~ Thomas Fuller

#36 Gallstones

The gallbladder is a small, pear-shaped pouch that is located behind the liver. Its main job is to save the cholesterol-rich bile that is secreted from the liver. Bile is important for digesting fatty foods. Many people, especially women and the elderly, have gallbladder problems, usually in the form of gallstones. Gallstones form if the bile contains high levels of cholesterol, which result when there isn't enough bile to saturate the cholesterol. For some people gallstones can be horribly painful, while for

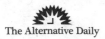

others they are asymptomatic. The conventional treatment of gallstones is usually to remove the gallbladder. Although surgery risks are low and result in pain relief, there is some inherent risk with any surgical procedure and some patients report ongoing digestive problems after removal.

There are a number of alternative actions that can be taken to alleviate gallstones, including ACV.

Application:

Before beginning an ACV flush for gallstones, you must drink ½ teaspoon of ACV with a 6-ounce glass of organic, unfiltered apple juice (if you have blood sugar issues, use filtered water instead) for three days, each morning when you wake up. Organic apple juice contains malic acid, potassium, pectins and enzymes which help cleanse the body and soften small gallstones. Also, cut back your fat, dairy and meat intake and eat plenty of apples and other fresh fruits and vegetables for about three days before the flush. For the flush, mix ⅓ parts organic olive oil with ⅔ parts unfiltered apple juice and 1 teaspoon of ACV. Drink this mixture 3 times a day on the first day. At night, sleep on your side with your right knee pulled towards your chest. On the second day, drink the mixture twice. Drink as much unfiltered apple juice as you would like during the flush, but nothing else, not even water.

It is possible that you may feel sick during the flush as your body removes toxins, bile and mucus. If this happens, you can drink a couple of glasses of purified water until you empty your stomach.

Eat a large mixed salad with ACV and olive oil dressing on day three, and continue to slowly add back in more food. Eating as many whole foods as possible is recommended.

* Do not do this flush if you are diabetic unless you are supervised by a health professional.

#37 Anxiety

It rips through your body like a torpedo, tensing every nerve, pushing your adrenal glands into overdrive and robbing precious years from your life. Stress is no joke, and millions of Americans live their lives in such a heightened state of anxiety that their bodies no longer respond properly.

Anxiety is one of the most significant health issues of our century, to the extent that it is being called a global epidemic. Although being stressed is a normal and often healthy response, excessive stress can be disabling. This is sometimes referred to as "burnout," and millions of Americans are burning out on a daily basis.

To treat the ever-increasing problem of stress and anxiety, we have become a pill popping nation. Sales of anti-stress medications continue to rise, and a comprehensive global report on anxiety disorders forecasts that the market will reach almost 6 billion dollars by 2017.

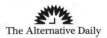

The sad fact is that the response rate to pharmacological treatment protocols is shaky at best. Over one third of people taking anti-anxiety medications do not respond to drugs, and many of these drugs carry significant side effects that counter any positives they deliver.

So, what are we to do about all this pent-up stress that is crippling our lives? The solution, many health experts feel, can be found in safe and effective natural therapies, including the use of ACV.

ACV breaks down proteins into amino acids, which fuel the process of hormone production. In addition to growth hormone, tryptophan is also created. This hormone helps to release serotonin, the "feel-good" neurotransmitter that eases tension and helps us relax.

Application

Mix a glass of warm water with 2 teaspoons of pure honey and 1 tablespoon of apple cider vinegar. Sip throughout the day. Be sure to cut out processed and refined foods and eat plenty of fresh foods, including fruits and vegetables and healthy fats such as grass fed beef and coconut oil.

DID YOU KNOW: The Following Herbs have Anti-Anxiety Properties

Valerian root, also referred to as nature's Valium, has been used for centuries as a natural way to relieve anxiety, insomnia and tense muscles. This natural herb can be sedating for some, so it's best to use it before bed when trying it out for the first time.

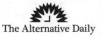
The Alternative Daily

Passion flower is a great remedy for those with mild to moderate anxiety, although it may still be useful for people with severe anxiety issues. This natural herb is known for reducing tension, calming the mind and preventing agitation.

Hops are commonly used for general nervousness, and are also effective for quieting the mind. This particular herb is great for someone who has a hard time falling asleep at night, or just needs to calm down during stressful times.

Skullcap is a powerful relaxant that can be used to eliminate nervous tension in those with severe anxiety. It is used as a sedative and muscle relaxant, and also helps to fight insomnia. While the effects are similar to valerian root, they are more pronounced.

Motherwort is an effective, yet gentle, way to ease stress, tension and anxiety. Many pregnant women favor this herb because it can be safely used in the third trimester to eliminate stress and stimulate circulation. Motherwort is also effective at inducing calmness without causing fatigue.

#38 Jellyfish Stings

Jellyfish are beautiful sea creatures that are fun to watch from a distance, but no fun to step on. Because they are often washed onto shore, a great many people are stung each year. A jellyfish sting is painful and itchy, especially if tentacles are left in the skin. A sting from a box jellyfish can even be fatal. According to the *Medical Journal of Australia*, ACV helps to cut the pain, reduce the toxic insult of the sting and also prevents the release of more venom.

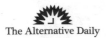

Application:

Keep a small jar of cotton pads soaked in ACV with you when you visit the beach. If you are stung, apply a cotton pad to the sting site immediately, and continue to apply freshly soaked pads until pain and swelling decrease.

Note: Seek immediate medical attention if your breathing becomes impaired, if you experience major swelling or exhibit other signs of a severe allergic reaction.

#39 Cuts

To stop the bleeding of minor cuts, soak a cotton ball in 1 ounce of ACV. Place on the affected area and repeat 3 times a day to speed healing.

#40 Dizziness

Help control minor dizziness by mixing 1 tablespoon of ACV and 2 tablespoons of pure honey in 8 ounces of warm distilled water. Drink this 3 times a day. For cases of intense dizziness, see your medical practitioner. Do not consume this mixture if you are diabetic.

 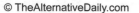

#41 Cellulite

To smooth stubborn areas of cellulite, mix 3 parts ACV with one part massage oil and massage the area daily. You can also drink 2 table-spoons of ACV in 8 ounces of water on an empty stomach each morning.

DID YOU KNOW: Over 80 percent of women develop cellulite at some point in their lives.

#42 Conjunctivitis

To relieve the pain and itchiness of conjunctivitis, mix 1 teaspoon of ACV with 4 teaspoons of filtered water. Moisten a clean cotton ball and wipe around the eyes 3 times a day. Discard each cotton ball when done. Do not pour the solution directly into the eyes.

#43 Impetigo

To relieve the soreness associated with impetigo, mix 1 ounce of ACV with 4 ounces of water and use the mixture to moisten a clean cotton ball. Apply to the infected area 3 times daily.

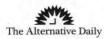

#44 Insomnia

A new study performed by the Brigham and Women's Hospital (BWH) has associated certain symptoms of insomnia with a significantly higher risk of dying from cardiovascular disease.

This study was rather large in scale, following 23,000 men with self-reported insomnia over a six-year time period. The researchers documented deaths and causes of death during this time, and compared them to the reported insomnia symptoms.

After results were adjusted for factors including lifestyle, other chronic illnesses and age, they showed that the men who reported having a difficult time falling asleep had a 55 percent higher risk of death related to cardiovascular disease, compared to men who did not have this insomnia symptom.

The researchers also found that the men who reported "non-restorative" sleep had a 32 percent higher risk of death from cardiovascular disease-related factors than men who did not have this issue.

The study's senior author, Dr. Xiang Gao, says, "we know that sleep is important for cardiovascular health and many studies have linked poor or insufficient sleep with increased risk factors for cardiovascular-related diseases. Now we know that not only can poor sleep impact disease risk, but it may also impact our longevity."

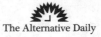

Dr. Gao continues, "while further research is necessary to confirm these findings, there is overwhelming evidence that practicing good sleep hygiene and prioritizing sufficient and restful sleep is an often overlooked but important modifiable risk factor in overall health."

While the benefits of sleep, and the risks of not getting quality sleep, are innumerable and relatively well known, getting a good night's sleep can be very difficult for some individuals, especially those prone to stress. Luckily, there are many time-tested natural methods available to aid us in getting proper shut-eye. Before reaching for an over-the-counter or prescription sleep aid, try this easy-to-make ACV tonic.

Application:

To calm your mind and body before bed, mix 1 tablespoon ACV with 8 ounces of warm water. If you like, add a teaspoon or so of raw honey. Drink a glass before you retire for the night. If you find yourself waking during the night you can drink another glass to help you fall back asleep.

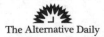

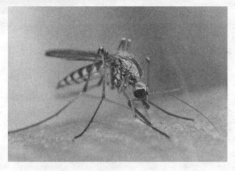

#45 Mosquito Bites

Ouch... the awful, pesky sting of a mosquito is not something anyone enjoys. Mosquitoes are blood-sucking insects that know how to spoil a good party. Sure, you can spray yourself with toxic bug repel-lant and they may stay away for a while, but who wants the worry of all of those dangerous chemicals?

The good news is that there are natural, safe and effective ways to keep mosquitoes at bay so that you can enjoy your outdoor living space all summer long. Try any one of these five natural solutions, or combine them for best protection.

Make Your Own Bug-be-Gone Spray

Add distilled water to an empty (and clean) spray bottle to the halfway mark.

- Fill the spray bottle until it is almost full with witch hazel.
- Add 2 tablespoons ACV
- Add 60 drops of essential oils and shake well. Use rosemary, clove or eucalyptus.

Make Your Garden Mosquito-Proof

- Plant citronella, rosemary, catnip, mint, marigolds, basil, lemon-grass and garlic. Mosquitoes hate the smell of these plants, and they will stay away.

- Dump out any sitting water, and avoid leaving things out that would collect water. Keep animal dishes and birdbaths clean and fresh.

- Mosquitoes love damp, dark places; keep those places to a minimum by keeping up with your garden. Weed, trim bushes, and keep the lawn mowed. Not only will it look nice, but you will reduce your mosquito population substantially.

- Put up plenty of bird houses, especially a purple martin house. Birds eat hundreds of mosquitoes each day, and will also be a pleasant addition to your landscape.

If you happen to get stung by a mosquito, reach for some ACV. Not only will the vinegar bring instant itch relief, it will also work to reduce inflammation and pain.

Application

Mix 1 tablespoon of ACV with 1 cup of water and apply to the sting with a soft and clean cotton pad. Repeat as many times as necessary to reduce swelling and pain.

"The art of medicine consists of amusing the patient while Nature cures the disease." ~Voltaire

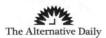

#46 Asthma

Some people who use inhalers for asthma report much relief when they use ACV. This method should only be used when your breathing is not severely compromised. ACV may help relax bronchial passages. Soak a cotton pad in ½ cup of ACV and breathe it in slowly and deeply. You can also sip on a mixture of 1 tablespoon of ACV mixed in 8 ounces of filtered water.

#47 Canker Sores

Canker sores are very small in size, but they can cause a tremendous amount of pain. The cause of canker sores remain unknown, but over 20 percent of the population suffers from them. Canker sores can be simple or complex. Simple cankers appear a few times a year, while complex sores are less common.

It is thought that canker sores may stem from stress, injury or an over-intake of citrus foods. A weakened immune system, gastrointestinal disease or nutritional problems may also trigger complex canker sores.

Symptoms of severe canker sores range from painful burning or tingling to fever, fatigue and even swelling of the lymph nodes. While the pain of a canker sore may last for seven to ten days, the sore may take up to three weeks to fully disappear.

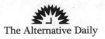

The Alternative Daily

Conventional treatments for canker sores include rinses and ointments, or you can try a more natural approach which includes ACV, that is effective due to its antibacterial and anti-inflammatory properties.

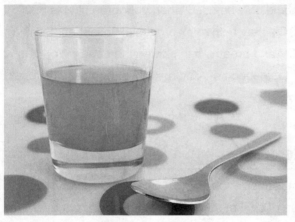

Application

Mouth Rinse: Add 1 teaspoon of ACV to 4 ounces of water. Rinse your mouth, being sure to allow the solution to pass over the canker sore. Do this several times a day until the canker sore disappears.

Calcium Magnesium Wash: Mix a teaspoon of apple cider vinegar into 8 ounces of warm water, and add a teaspoon of calcium-magnesium powder. Fill up the remaining portion of the glass with cold water and sip on the drink.

#48 Inflammation

The word "inflammation" comes from the Latin word "inflammo," which means, "I set alight, I ignite." It has been called the "root of all disease," and consists of a natural bodily reaction gone very bad. When the body is threatened by something harmful, such as damaged cells, pathogens or irritants, there is an immediate biological response to try to remove the

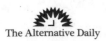

harmful stimulus and promote healing. Contrary to what you may think, inflammation does not mean infection, even if an infection is what caused the inflammation in the first place.

At first, inflammation is beneficial and highly protective. If you cut your finger, your body stimulates an acute inflammatory response to protect the wound and hasten healing.

What is dangerous is inflammation in the body caused by poor diet, stress, menopause, environmental issues and injuries that have never been addressed. Studies have shown that inflammation in the body can contribute to or cause diseases such as cancer, autoimmune diseases including lupus, rheumatoid arthritis, Crohn's disease, psoriasis, irritable bowel syndrome, diabetes, allergies, arthritis, atherosclerosis and Alzheimer's, as well as heart disease.

Making lifestyle changes such as switching to an anti-inflammatory diet, exercise and stress reduction can all help to reduce inflammation gone awry. Our modern diets are loaded with refined sugars and processed foods, all of which contribute to chronic low-grade inflammation. Switching to a whole food diet that includes plenty of fruits and vegetables, along with healthy fats from grass fed meats and tropical oils such a coconut oil, can significantly reduce inflammation.

In addition to making lifestyle changes, ACV contains natural anti-inflammatory properties and is a great addition to an anti-inflammatory lifestyle.

Application

Mix 2 tablespoons of ACV with a glass of filtered water and drink it 3 times a day during meals. You can also add ACV liberally to salads, or drizzle on other veggie dishes.

Perfect at-home pedicure: Want to skip the expensive spa pedicures? Try an at-home variety using ACV. Simply pour 1 cup of ACV into a bowl of warm water to soothe your tired, achy feet. This is perfect if you are on your feet at lot, or wear shoes with little support. Add 10 drops of peppermint essential oil for an invigorating soak.

#49 Heavy Metal Poisoning

Let's face it, we are exposed to an alarming amount of toxins on a daily basis. From the BPA that lines your canned goods to the pesticides liberally sprayed on anything alive these days, our bodies are constantly absorbing an outrageous amount of chemicals.

Even though you may try to live as pure a life as possible, sneaky sources of dangerous metals are everywhere, even in the so-called "all natural" products that fool consumers into believing their ingredients are safe.

Over time, high concentrations of metals build up in our systems and can lead to a wide variety of conditions, including, but not limited to:

- Anemia
- Dizziness
- Fatigue

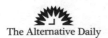

- Dry skin
- Joint or muscle aches
- Loss of appetite
- Low blood pressure
- Nausea
- Vitamin and mineral deficiencies

Try as you may, there's just no getting around the obscene amounts of toxins we are exposed to daily. But that doesn't mean you are forced to live with theses conditions. There are many ways to rid yourself of heavy metal accumulation, including drinking more water, consuming more whole foods and exercising daily. Apple cider vinegar is often referred to as a "natural chelator," due to its exceptional ability to help the body detoxify.

Application

Mix 2 tablespoons of apple cider vinegar with 8 ounces of distilled water and drink 3 times a day during a prescribed detox program.

DID YOU KNOW: A large number of dangerous toxins are found in everyday items such as carpets, electronics, pillows, appliances and furniture.

#50 Depression

Depression is a serious condition that can affect every aspect of life, as sufferers well know. The National Alliance on Mental Illness estimates that depression affects over 15 million American adults today, and this does not even include the numerous adolescents that show depression symptoms.

In an attempt to lift the weight of depression and try to lead normal lives, many people turn to prescription antidepressants. However, antidepressants often do more harm than good, as they lead to an array of side effects, some of which may actually worsen the depression by creating new emotional imbalances. Before turning to dangerous drugs, try the natural approach first – you may be surprised at the positive results.

Some research shows that niacin, also known as vitamin B3, can alleviate depression in many cases. Many people suffering from depression have been found to have very low niacin levels. Studies have also shown that high stress levels, poor diet and lack of sleep can cause depression and anxiety. Improper functioning of the liver and digestive tract can also trigger depression.

Apple cider vinegar can detoxify and regulate the pH of the body while supporting healthy liver and kidney function. In addition, when you take ACV before meals it helps to break down proteins into amino acids. As mentioned earlier, these amino acids fuel hormone production in the body, including the creation of tryptophan. Tryptophan in turn helps release

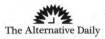

serotonin that elevates mo

at bay. This is especially i

of sunlight have a negati

people who suffer from §

benefit from ACV.

Application

Take 1 tablespoon of

minutes prior to each .

The Apple Cider Vinegar Miracle
81 Ways to Naturally Cleanse Your Body & House a

#52 Hair

Many people a

men are the

experien

Hair

#51 Hot Flashes

While some hormonal conditions may cause hot flashes, the majority are the result of menopause. For many perimenopausal and menopausal women, hot flashes are an annoying reality that can often interrupt sleep and leave one uncomfortable and irritable.

Many naturopaths recommend ACV to patients seeking relief from hot flashes. To reduce the uncomfortableness of hot flashes, mix 2 tablespoons of ACV into 8 ounces of filtered warm water and drink 2 times a day, morning and evening. You can add a teaspoon of stevia for a sweeter mixture.

DID YOU KNOW: Excess sugar, processed meat and dairy can trigger hot flashes. Stick to a whole food diet with plenty of organic fruits and veggies, as well as healthy fats from olive and coconut oils.

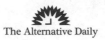

The Alternative Daily

LOSS

e under the impression that when it comes to hair loss,
only ones affected. However, there are many women who
e it too.

oss can be a symptom of a short term event, such as extreme
ess, pregnancy, medication or disease; in these situations the hair
normally grows back following the end of the event.

One in four women experience female pattern baldness. These women lose their hair for many of the same reasons as men. The hormone DHT is at least partially to blame, and heredity is a significant factor.

One of the first things you should do if you're experiencing hair loss is to take a look at your lifestyle. Are you eating a healthy, balanced diet filled with plenty of organic fruits and vegetables, healthy fats like coconut oil and olive oil, and proteins derived from lean meats, nuts, seeds and legumes? It's also important to avoid eating processed foods or any other

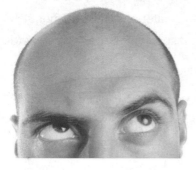

foods laden with chemicals. A poor diet can have a significant negative impact on hair growth.

Be sure to incorporate daily physical activity and stress-relieving practices into your day, such as deep-breathing or meditation.

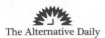

In addition, there are a number of herbs and natural therapies that can help to rejuvenate your hair, including ACV. Good blood circulation is essential for a healthy scalp and strong hair. This vinegar helps to increase circulation of blood to the hair roots, which strengthens these roots and even promotes growth. If you use a number of commercial products on your hair it is likely that your hair's pH balance is off. Using ACV on your hair will restore and maintain this balance, which creates an optimum environment for hair growth. In addition, the antifungal and anti-bacterial properties of ACV help to keep bacteria, dandruff and other skin conditions that may promote hair loss, at bay.

Application

Mix 4 tablespoons of ACV into a 4 ounce glass of water. Add 12 drops of rosemary or lemon essential oil and shake well. Massage the mixture into your scalp and let it set for 20 minutes before rinsing it out with cold water.

TRY IT: Herbs that Stimulate Hair Growth

Rosemary Oil

Rosemary essential oil has been used for centuries by many cultures to stimulate hair growth. It stimulates circulation to the scalp and destroys any bacteria that could clog hair follicles. As an added bonus, it can also make your hair more shiny.

Lavender Essential Oil

Lavender essential oil is also known to be quite effective for rejuvenating hair. A study by a group of dermatologists in Scotland showed that 44 percent of patients who had suffered from hair loss experienced new hair growth when they massaged their scalp daily with lavender and other essential oils for seven months.

Clary Sage Oil

Hormones are an important issue when it comes to hair loss and growth. Clary sage is known to promote estrogen balance and prevent thickening in the membrane tissue around the hair follicle which creates hair loss.

Using Essential Oils

Start by using a cleansing shampoo, one which is designed to remove buildup of chemicals, grease or chlorine in your hair and scalp. Alternatively, you can mix about two tablespoons of baking soda into your regular shampoo and follow with a vinegar rinse by combining 1 tablespoon of apple cider vinegar with 1 cup of cold water.

Mix the above oils, using five drops of each, and gently massage in small circular motions all over your scalp. You can use this as an overnight treatment or just leave on as long as possible and then shampoo it out. Adding five drops of each of these oils to your organic shampoo each time you wash your hair can also help.

Have patience – it does take time and effort to encourage healthier hair, but the potential rewards of a shiny, full head of hair are well worth it!

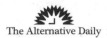

#53 Heart Health

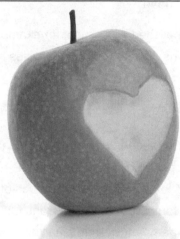

Good heart health is essential for the prevention of all types of heart disease, including cardiovascular and coronary heart disease, as well as stroke.

Many other health disorders are related to heart, arterial and circulatory health, including dysfunction in organs that are fed by our arteries and veins. These include conditions like impotence, brain diseases and dementia, macular degeneration and more.

Just a century ago, heart disease was so rare that it had only been just discovered, but today, it is our number one killer, responsible for more than 40 percent of all deaths worldwide. Taking steps to improve and support good heart health is a must for longevity, as well as for quality of life.

One of the most important things you can do for your heart is to be active. Aerobic exercise is essential for managing cardiovascular risk. It helps control your weight and also decreases the chances of developing other conditions that can put a strain on your heart, such as diabetes and high blood pressure. It also helps to reduce stress and lower inflammation, both of which can contribute to heart disease.

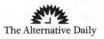

The Alternative Daily

Most health experts believe that getting 30 to 60 minutes of moderately intense physical activity on most days of the week is optimal, but even lesser amounts can offer benefits to the heart.

Your exercise doesn't have to be accomplished all at once; for example, it can be broken up into 10-minute sessions. Remember that activities like doing household chores and gardening also count toward your total.

Avoid Processed Foods and All Trans Fats

Avoiding all processed foods is optimal for supporting good heart health, but staying away from any and all hydrogenated oils, also known as trans fats, is essential. These oils are thought to be responsible for much of the increase in heart disease over the past four decades or so. Trans fats are harmful to the body, and particularly to the heart, even in small amounts.

If you see anything that says partially hydrogenated (oil) as an ingredient, stay away. Using organic, cold-pressed olive oil and coconut oil offers heart healthy benefits that can help lower bad cholesterol and reduce buildup on arterial walls.

Good Nutrition

Eating a heart-healthy diet includes consuming plenty of organic fruits and vegetables, as well as foods that contain healthy fats like nuts and seeds, wild-caught salmon, coconut and olive oils.

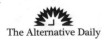

Eating onions regularly can also help to keep the blood from forming clots, and even to dissolve those that exist in the circulatory system. Drinking a moderate amount of alcohol, preferably red wine, can also protect the heart. It's suggested that men consume no more than two drinks per day, while women should stick to one.

In order to continue beating, the heart must have a constant supply of of power and energy. Can we change to ACV helps make the heart stronger while normalizing blood pressure and cholesterol. while normalizing blood pressure and cholesterol. Recent studies indicate that ACV can even reduce arterial plaque.

Application

Mix one tablespoon ACV and 1 teaspoon raw honey in 8 ounces of warm water. Drink a glass of the mixture each morning and one hour before lunch and dinner. If you are a diabetic, use 2 drops of stevia to sweeten the drink instead of honey.

"When you arise in the morning, think of what a precious privilege it is to be alive - to breathe, to think, to enjoy, to love." ~Marcus Aurelius

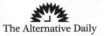

The Alternative Daily

#54 Bad Breath

Mouth bacteria doesn't just cause bad breath and lead to unhealthy teeth and gums – it's also linked to other health problems, such as heart disease and even dementia.

Plaque is a type of biofilm which consists of a thin grouping of bacteria living on the teeth and gum tissue. If allowed to build up, it can cause gum disease. Eventually, as the gum tissue pulls away from the teeth, the bacteria can destroy the bone underneath that supports the teeth, causing tooth loss.

Root causes of bad breath include bacteria hiding in teeth and below the gum line, as well as an improperly functioning digestive system.

FOODS THAT IMPROVE HEALTHY GUT BACTERIA AND FIGHT BAD BREATH

Garlic: While garlic may temporarily give you bad breath, its antimicrobial properties actually help to battle bacteria in the mouth. A compound found in garlic, known as allicin, helps to inhibit periodontitis, a serious gum infection that damages soft tissues and destroys the bone that supports the teeth. If you're concerned about its immediate effects, chewing a sprig of parsley can help to alleviate garlic breath.

Apples: Taking a big bite out of an apple and chewing on it actually helps to scrub your teeth clean. This fruit has a high concentration of malic acid, which is even used in some brands of toothpaste. This substance helps to increase saliva in the mouth, which cleans the teeth and helps to remove stains, according to a study out of the University of Grenada in Spain.

Pineapples: Eating pineapple isn't just a great way to take you to the tropics – it can actually help to whiten your teeth. Pineapples contain the enzyme bromelain, an anti-inflammatory agent that acts like a natural stain remover and helps to break up the plaque that builds up on your teeth. It's the only food found in nature that contains this enzyme.

Onions: Onions contain sulfur compounds and thiosulfinates, which are known to decrease bacteria. However, to get the antibacterial effect of these compounds, the onion must be eaten raw, as cooking will destroy them.

Ginger: Ginger is not only a delicious spice, it also offers potent anti-inflammatory properties that can support healthy mouth tissue. Periodontal disease is an inflammatory condition that may cause the loss of bone and supportive connective tissue. Using ginger to spice up your foods, or adding it to hot tea, helps to keep inflammation in check.

Carrots: Munching on raw carrots helps to stimulate saliva and can naturally cleanse the mouth. These brightly-colored veggies are also packed full of vitamin A, which is essential for healthy tooth enamel.

Cranberry Juice: A study published in the Journal of Antimicrobial Chemotherapy revealed that cranberry juice helps to stop the growth of the collection of bacteria that builds up on the teeth and throughout the mouth, causing tooth decay and periodontal disease. Just make sure you are using the juice from fresh cranberries; those cranberry juice cocktails at the supermarket are not nearly the same thing.

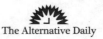

Organic Cheese: As cheese is rich in minerals like calcium, protein and phosphorous, it can help buffer the acids in the mouth. Calcium and phosphorous also help to build stronger bones and repair teeth.

Water: Drinking plenty of filtered or pure spring water each day offers a wealth of health benefits. One of these benefits is promoting saliva production, which helps to keep teeth white. Be sure to drink a glass of water during and after a meal to rinse your mouth free of loose plaque and other debris.

By enjoying the above-listed foods as part of a healthy diet, you'll increase your odds of having a natural, beautiful smile, without having to shell out hundreds or even thousands of dollars to get it!

In addition to eating healthy foods, you can make an easy, natural, homemade remedy for bad breath using ACV. Because ACV contains potent antibacterial properties, it can help to kill bacteria in the gums and teeth, as well as promote healthy gut bacteria.

Application

After you brush and floss your teeth, gargle with ½ tablespoon ACV and 1 cup of distilled water. Spit out the ACV mixture after you gargle and rinse with pure water. For healthy gut bacteria support, drink 1 tablespoon of ACV with 8 ounces of distilled water prior to each meal.

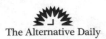

#55 Gout

Gout, a type of arthritis, is a painful condition that is caused by a buildup of uric acid in the blood. Most often the big toe, foot and ankle are compromised. This condition causes sudden burning pain, stiffness, swelling and redness. Attacks often come at night and can interrupt sleep. It can often take several weeks for the pain to go away.

Avoiding high-purine foods such as fish, organ meats, beef and shellfish, as well as alcohol, fatty fried foods, fructose and high-fat sauces can help keep attacks at bay. ACV alkalizes the pH balance of the blood, helps your body eliminate the buildup of uric acid and can relieve the pain and swelling associated with gout.

Application

You can also soak your affected area in a mixture of 1 cup ACV and enough water to cover. Immerse your feet in water for 5 minutes, remove and pat dry. Repeat this 2 times a day until the gout disappears. You can also drink a mixture of 2 tablespoons of ACV in 8 ounces of filtered water 3 times a day.

#56 Tired Eyes

If you work long hours in front of a computer or drive a lot, you may experience tired or sore eyes. Take 2 teaspoons of ACV mixed with 1 teaspoon of pure honey and 8 ounces of warm, filtered water 3 times a day.

#57 Hiccups

Have you ever had hiccups and not known how to get rid of them? Maybe you have tried holding your breath or even having a friend scare you. If these things aren't working for you, try ACV. Since hiccups are generally caused by either low stomach acid, slow digestion of protein or eating too much, ACV works great. ACV will help restore stomach acid balance and calm diaphragm spasms. Mix 2 tablespoons of ACV into 8 ounces of filtered water and drink when you have the hiccups. To prevent hiccups, drink this mixture before meals.

#58 Fibromyalgia

If you or someone you know suffers from fibromyalgia, then you know how frustrating this medical condition can be. Often misunderstood because of the large variance in symptoms, fibromyalgia is characterized by chronic and widespread musculoskeletal pain. Other common symptoms include fatigue, sleep problems, joint stiffness, anxiety, depression, dry eyes and mouth, headaches, dizziness, Raynaud's syndrome and cognitive impairment.

What Causes Fibromyalgia?

For the last twenty years, scientists have been struggling to find a cause for this somewhat mysterious disease. Various theories exist, including heavy metal toxicity, growth hormone deficiency, emotional trauma, bacterial infections, nutritional deficiencies and sleep dysfunction.

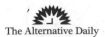

The latest findings reveal that fibromyalgia may be a central processing disorder. This means that when you have this condition, you experience an amplification in pain due to abnormal sensory processing in the central nervous system. So, those that suffer have a lower pain threshold because of an increased sensitivity to pain signals.

Triggers and Treatment

Fibromyalgia appears to be a condition of triggers. In other words, certain things may trigger onset. This may be an emotional trauma, infection, surgery, illness, or the development of another disorder such as lupus or rheumatoid arthritis. These triggers do not cause fibromyalgia, but awaken an already present abnormality.

Unfortunately, the most common approach to dealing with fibromyalgia has been to mask the symptoms with drugs that do very little more than pad the pockets of the drug companies. This approach is partly due to the misunderstanding of the condition, and partly thanks to our symptom-based medical system.

Diet

Many people who suffer from fibromyalgia experience a significant reduction in pain after eliminating certain foods from their diets. These foods include sugar, citrus, dairy, wheat and corn. While there is not a one-size-fits-all diet, it appears that eliminating all artificial sweeteners and the foods mentioned above makes a tremendous difference.

Emotional Issues

The Centers for Disease Control (CDC) states that over 855 of all diseases have some sort of emotional element. Those that suffer from fibromyalgia may be able to backtrack and identify a very stressful past event that might have triggered the illness. This could be an experience that caused great trauma.

Dealing with the trauma may provide the healing necessary to feel good again. Some professionals recommend Emotional Freedom Technique (EFT), which is like a needle-less acupuncture that you can even do on yourself at home. It is an easy technique to learn, and is used by people dealing with Post Traumatic Stress Disorder (PTSD) with great success.

Exercise

Exercise is beneficial for everyone, and is especially beneficial for those suffering from chronic pain. Although getting going may be hard, it will help reduce pain. A study done at Harvard University indicated that women who participated in moderately intense exercise found a relief in pain. They did a combination of stretching, walking and strength training. The average pain reduction was 45 percent in just 16 weeks.

It is important not to overdo it. The best form of exercise is gradual and consistent. Some people have found that exercising in warm water helps, as well as taking yoga or pilates classes. Jarring activities such as horse-back riding or running may do more harm than good.

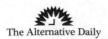

Massage

Everyone loves a good massage; it is one of the oldest forms of medical care used to treat pain. The health benefits of therapeutic massage are well documented. An article by CNN recently noted that fibromyalgia patients found great relief with massage. Massage increases endorphins that promote a sense of well being, helps boost attention, strengthens the immune system, reduces cortisol levels, relieves insomnia and reduces anxiety.

Sleep

Once you increase your activity level, it is easier to sleep. The National Fibromyalgia Research Association states that 75 percent of sufferers have sleep disturbances and fatigue. Poor sleep definitely makes symptoms worse. If you don't get a good night's sleep, your immune system is compromised, and you feel groggy.

Enhancing sleep is a critical part of the overall natural treatment approach to dealing with fibromyalgia. To help get the best night's rest possible, avoid late night snacks, avoid alcohol, listen to a white noise CD, sleep in complete darkness, establish a regular bedtime and wake time, keep your bedroom cool, wear socks to bed, avoid caffeine after lunch, take a warm bath or sauna before bed and keep all electronics out of the bedroom.

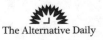
The Alternative Daily

Apple cider vinegar helps to stimulate digestion and proper pancreas function. It also helps to restore the body's acid and alkaline balance, and relieves joint pain and inflammation associated with fibromyalgia.

Application

Mix an ACV tonic by combining 2 table-spoons of ACV and 8 ounces of filtered water. Drink this 3 times a day. Add some raw honey or stevia for sweetener and drink warm or cold.

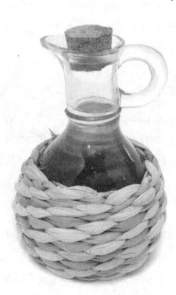

"Everything in food works together to create health or disease. The more we think that a single chemical characterizes a whole food, the more we stray into idiocy."
~ T. Colin Campbell, The China Study

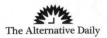

Around the Home and Garden

Not only is ACV a great remedy for many health conditions, it is also a trusty companion to have around your home. Here are just a few of the many things you can do with it:

#59 General Cleaning

For clean toilets and a fresh-smelling bathroom, pour some ACV into your toilet and allow it to sit overnight. You can also use it in your dishwasher instead of detergent. Clean microwaves, windows, glasses, wood and tile floors and mirrors with a mixture of ½ cup apple cider vinegar and 1 cup water.

#60 Unclog Drains

Commercial drain cleaners are dangerous and can cause stinging of the eyes, rashes, respiratory damage and other medical conditions. To avoid this, use a mixture of ACV and baking soda. This solution is not only better for your health, but also better for your pipes. To unclog drains, funnel ½ cup of baking soda into your drain and follow it with 1 cup of apple cider vinegar. After the foaming stops, flush the drain with hot water and wait five minutes. After this, flush with cold water. If you have a slow drain, you can pour in ½ cup of salt followed by 2 cups of boiling apple cider vinegar, then flush with hot water, followed by cold water. Do this monthly to keep your drains running smoothly.

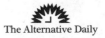
The Alternative Daily

#61 Remove Fridge Odors

If you are hit with a knock-down odor every time you open your fridge, you may want to consider a good cleaning with an ACV and water mixture. Simply place equal amounts of each in a spray bottle and clean away. When you are finished, set a small, shallow cup of ACV in the fridge in a location where it won't get knocked over. It will continue to freshen your fridge for up to a month.

#62 Clean Gold Jewelry

Don't buy expensive jewelry cleaners when you can simply soak your rings and other shiny things in a small cup of ACV. Soak jewelry for twenty minutes, rinse with warm water and dry with a soft cloth. You will be amazed at how new your jewelry looks.

#63 Fruit Fly Destroyer

If you have ever battled fruit flies, you know how much of a nuisance they can be. Pour some ACV into a container with a few holes and watch the flies disappear.

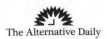

#64 Removing Smoke Odor

Smoke gets trapped in things such as carpets and floors, but did you know that it gets trapped in walls, as well? To remove stale tobacco smells from your walls, wash them with a 50/50 mixture of ACV and water. After they dry, you should notice a huge difference in the odor, and your walls will sparkle.

#65 Remove Water Rings from Furniture

To remove the white rings left by wet glasses, mix equal parts of ACV and olive oil, and apply the mixture to your furniture with a soft cloth. Use another clean cloth for shining - being sure to go with the wood grain.

#66 Fleas and Ticks

ACV is useful for treating fleas and ticks on pets. Adding one part apple cider vinegar to one part water and spraying the mixture on your pet will help keep the pesky critters at bay. Be sure to saturate the entire coat, and repeat a few times a week during heavy flea season.

#67 Preserve Cut Flowers

To keep your beautiful garden bouquet looking its best, add 2 teaspoons of sugar and 2 teaspoons of ACV to your flower water. You can change this twice a week for perky and happy flowers.

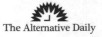

The Alternative Daily

#68 Kill Weeds

Steer clear of commercial weed killers, as they contain dangerous chemicals. Try spraying undiluted ACV directly onto weeds to keep them under control. This works great between patio stones or along edging.

#69 Improve Garden Soil

ACV helps soil to release iron, which is essential for healthy plant growth. Place 1 cup of ACV in a gallon of water and add to your garden beds. If you have plants that like acidic soil, such as azaleas, gardenias and rhododendrons, they will benefit greatly from this application.

#70 Clean Patios

To clean the dirt and mold that can build up between patio stones, use straight ACV and a strong, bristled brush. Rinse with a hose when done, and you will have a new-looking patio that will also discourage mold growth.

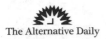

#71 Chicken Health

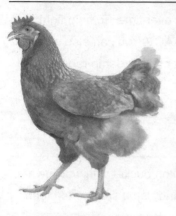

If you keep backyard chickens, there are many ways that you can use ACV in and around the coop. For starters, you can add a couple of tablespoons of ACV to your chicken waterers on a weekly basis. Be sure to do this only in plastic watering containers, not metal. Adding the vinegar to the water will help keep your chickens' respiratory and digestive systems healthy while keeping bacteria at bay and boosting immunity. If you want your eggs to sparkle, dip them in warm ACV. If you really love your chickens, you will give them a nice bubble bath from time to time, which will keep their feathers and skin healthy and bacteria-free. Just mix a few tablespoons of ACV with a gentle pet shampoo for the bath. Spray some ACV in and around the coop area to keep pests at bay. When it comes time to clean your waterers and feeders, add some ACV to your dishwater. This will help decontaminate and leave your containers sparkly clean.

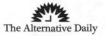
The Alternative Daily

#72 Dishwasher Refresher

Dishwashers, like all appliances, start to smell over time. To help fight dishwasher odors, run an empty load with just ACV. You can also wipe down the inside and outside of your dishwasher with a damp rag sprayed with ACV.

#73 Mildew Remover

For mildew in and around the home, fill a 5 gallon bucket with warm water and add 2 cups of ACV. Mix the solution well and use a sponge to clean the area.

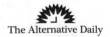

Keys to Aging Gracefully

"He who is of a calm and happy nature will hardly feel the pressure of age, but to him who is of an opposite disposition, youth and age are equally a burden." ~Plato (427-346 B.C.)

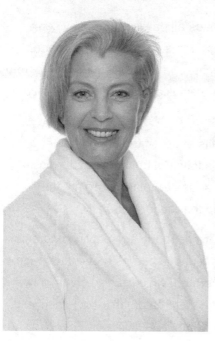

Longevity is big business in America today — the dream that anything is possible, even reversing our internal clocks, drives millions of people to seek out sometimes drastic measures to reduce the signs of aging. Plastic surgery, botox and other invasive procedures bring high dollar and high risk.

The key to fighting aging does not rest in some procedure, injection, pill, or even our makeup, but rather on achieving internal balance. The overall health of the body determines how gracefully we age.

The human body has a unique way of achieving a healthy internal balance no matter how old we are. The key to unlocking the anti-aging code rests in providing the raw materials that we need for cellular repair and restoration.

Foods that Restore Balance

Whole foods bring balance to the body and supply energy, while processed foods create unhealthy internal chaos and rob us of our youth. Here are five anti-aging foods to add to your diet today.

Carrots: Eat organic carrots as you please all day long, or enjoy some freshly-juiced carrots. These little orange gems contain beta-carotene, which slows down aging, and also vitamin A, which prevents damage from too many UVB rays and stops premature wrinkles in their tracks. It also helps to balance out skin tone.

Green Tea: The well-researched benefits of green tea are no longer a secret in America. Enjoying a cup of this flavorful tea on a regular basis will fight damaging free radicals. While stress accelerates aging, the amino acids contained in green tea help to reduce stress.

Berries: Fresh or frozen, berries have tremendous age-defying characteristics. Studies indicate that compounds found in berries prevent damage from oxidation. Mulberries contain resveratrol, which is also commonly found in wine. This substance is an anti-inflammatory that fights cancer and protects the body from free radical damage.

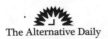

Aloe Vera: You can consume aloe vera internally in order to help the skin hydrate, or you can apply it topically and it will act as an exfoliant. Aloe contains an impressive list of compounds, including 96 percent water, 4 percent amino acids, minerals, enzymes, vitamins A, C and E as well as antioxidants, zinc and superoxide dismutases that are excellent for the skin.

Kiwis: Vitamin C is a powerful force against wrinkles, as it is necessary for the production of collagen. Although you can get vitamin C from many sources, kiwis have one of the highest concentrations of any fruit. Enjoy a kiwi each day for healthier and more vital skin.

Herbs Fight Oxidative Stress

Herbs are jam-packed full of natural, protective antioxidants and other properties that combat oxidative stress and reduce the signs and symptoms of aging. Here are three you don't want to miss.

Milk Thistle: Milk thistle is an ancient herb that has been recognized for its medicinal qualities for thousands of years. The extract is made from the plant's seeds, and contains 20 percent fatty acids and 80 percent silymarin, a powerful antioxidant. The fatty acids maintain cell membrane integrity and healthy cellular metabolism. Silymarin and its active compound, silybin, provide a strong defense against toxins while strengthening cell walls and blocking the free radicals responsible for signs of aging from attacking healthy cells. Milk thistle is often used topically to clean and protect the face from bacteria and toxins. As an oral supplement, milk thistle cleanses the liver and encourages the production of antioxidants that fight aging.

Ginger: Ginger is a potent anti-aging herb, mainly due to its anti-inflammatory properties. If sore or stiff joints are a concern, ginger goes right to work to alleviate the pain and inflammation. Ginger boosts the immune system and helps the body to absorb nutrients from the food we eat. Ginger contains over 50 different antioxidants that work at neutralizing free radicals in our bodies and stimulating the healing process in damaged cells. Ginger improves skin elasticity, prevents fine lines under eyes, and reduces forehead wrinkles and sagging skin. Make a tea with a teaspoon of ginger daily for best results.

Neem Oil: Both neem oil and neem leaves have been used to treat the skin for thousands of years. The neem tree belongs to the Mahogany family, and is an evergreen found mostly in India, Southeast Asia and parts of Africa. All parts of the tree, including the oils, seeds, bark and leaves, have health promoting qualities.

Neem oil is loaded with nutrients and contains a high level of antioxidants that protect the skin from environmental toxins. The oil is high in fatty acids and vitamin E, which are easily absorbed into the skin to help rejuvenate tired cells, restore elasticity and give skin a healthy glow. Aspirin-like properties soothe inflammation and irritation while fighting off bacteria.

Coconut Oil

A discussion about anti-aging would not be complete without mention of one of the most potent superfoods on the planet. Coconuts and their oil have been used by Pacific Islanders for thousands of years, both as a food source and a medicinal aid. It is a natural oil that is rich in

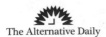

health-promoting lauric acid. According to the Coconut Research Center, "coconut helps to protect the body from harmful free radicals that promote premature aging and degenerative disease." Coconut oil softens skin, diminishes fine lines and wrinkles, and when taken internally, helps balance hormones and metabolism and improves immune function.

Don't Forget About Water

You lose about 8 glasses of water each day through your skin, and this water needs to be regularly replenished. Hydration is essential to overall health and wellness. It helps remove toxins, circulates nutrients through the body and reduces fine lines and wrinkles. Begin each day with a glass of warm lemon water.

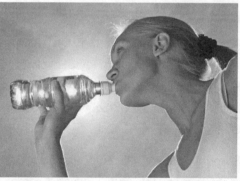

Lemons provide a valuable dose of vitamin C, which boosts immune function and helps the skin to repair itself. The potassium in lemons also helps keep free radicals at bay. Drink water freely throughout the day to stay hydrated.

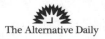
The Alternative Daily

Loving Your Skin

Skin is the largest organ of the body; we often fail to recognize this. Like all other organs, it needs to be well fed and nourished so that it can do its job. Healthy skin starts on the inside, with a good wholesome diet and plenty of pure water. Internal balance has a direct reflection on our skin, and if things are amiss on the interior, the exterior is not going to look so hot.

So, once you have your diet under control, you can turn your focus to the exterior. Skin is not the same as your pots and pans - it does not need to be scoured to be clean. In fact, heavy scouring of the skin can leave it dry and damaged. Instead, a healthy skin regimen should focus on gently removing dead skin cells, nourishing and moisturising.

An old understanding of the skin was that it was an impenetrable barrier, a shield of sorts that would not allow anything to enter or exit the body. However, now we know that while the skin does provide protection, it is not impenetrable. For example, if you stay soaking in the tub long enough, your skin starts to wrinkle.

Samuel Epstein, MD, author of *Toxic Beauty,* states that the skin readily takes in many things with which it comes into contact. There are a number of factors that come into play when considering what the skin will absorb, including skin health, hair, temperature and hydration ability.

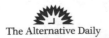

The Extension Toxicology Network (EXTOXNET) states that "chemicals can be absorbed through the skin and into the bloodstream, causing toxic effects." Similar information is found in the *Chemical Hazards Handbook* produced by the London Hazards Center Trust. It states, "although the skin acts as a protective barrier against many microorganisms and chemicals, some chemicals can penetrate the skin and enter the bloodstream."

As of today, our government does not require health studies or any pre-market testing of the chemicals in personal care products, even though we are 'eating' them on a daily basis through our skin. According to the Office of Cosmetics and Colors at the FDA, a cosmetic manufacturer can use almost any raw material in the making of a product without approval.

The cosmetic industry in the US is on its own to self-police using a Cosmetics Ingredient Review Board. This board has only rejected 11 ingredients for being unsafe. This is in comparison to the European Union, which has banned hundreds of ingredients.

To keep your skin healthy, it is imperative to only put on it that which you would be willing and able to ingest. ACV is a safe and effective substance that when used properly, can help keep your skin clean, bacteria-free and healthy.

Because ACV contains antibacterial and antifungal properties and can balance the skin's pH, it is an effective, toxicity-free way to keep your skin looking and feeling its best. In addition, ACV contains alpha hydroxy acids, which help to remove dead skin cells. People who commonly suffer from acne, dry or oily skin will find that their skin is much more balanced when using ACV, with fewer breakouts.

Here are just a few great ways to use ACV for great-looking and healthy skin:

#74 Facial Mask

To make a nourishing facial mask, mix equal parts of apple cider vinegar and bentonite clay, and add 1 tablespoon of raw honey. Apply to the skin. Leave on the detoxifying mask for about 10-15 minutes, rinse with warm water and pat dry. Repeat this once a week for best results.

#75 Face Wash

For a general, everyday face wash that will leave your skin feeling fresh, start by mixing 1 tablespoon of ACV with 3 tablespoons of warm water. Once your skin becomes accustomed to the ACV, you can change the mixture to a 2 to 1 ratio, and even to a 1 to 1 ratio if necessary. Apply the ACV wash to an inconspicuous part of your face using a clean cotton ball. Leave it on your skin for about one hour to be sure that you don't have a reaction. If you have a reaction you can further dilute the mixture, otherwise apply to the rest of your face and neck in upward sweeping motions. Rinse with warm water, pat dry and follow with an organic moisturizer.

Note: Make a larger batch and store it in a glass container for easy access.

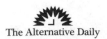

Customize it: Customize your facial wash by adding a few drops of tea tree or lavender essential oil. You can also infuse the water with fresh herbs; simply bring the water and herbs to a boil and simmer for 30 minutes. Once the water is cool, strain the herbs and add the ACV. Store in a clean glass jar with a lid.

#76 All Over Skin pH Balancer

Treat your whole body to an ACV wash by filling a small wash basin with warm water and ½ cup of ACV. Dip your hands in the mixture and massage all over your body until thoroughly wet. Apply this solution in the shower or bathtub so that you do not get the floor wet. Massage the balancer into your skin until it is dry; do not wash off. As an alternative, pour the mixture into a spray bottle and spray yourself after your shower or bath for an invigorating pH balancer.

#77 Facial Steam

To open up pores and help reduce the signs of aging, try an ACV wrinkle steamer. Simply mix 2 ounces of ACV with 1 quart of water and 1 sprig of fresh rosemary. Heat the water and ACV until hot and add the rosemary sprig. Pour into a shallow bowl and lower your head over the bowl (be careful not to touch the water). Cover your head with a towel and breathe in deeply while your skin is refreshed and cleansed. Pat your face with a clean towel and apply an organic skin moisturizer.

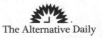

Dangers of Conventional Cosmetics

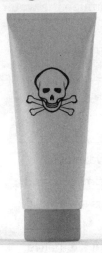

What did you have for lunch? Perhaps an apple, a nice salad with veggies and raw eggs, a little lead and a little hydrous magnesium silicate? You say what? If you have on makeup or any other conventional skincare products, we would say it is like you ate the dangerous chemicals that they contain. In fact, anything you put on your skin is as good as eaten!

According to a survey conducted by the Environmental Working Group, 25 percent of women use more than 15 products each day that contain over 126 different ingredients,

Here are just a few things that you may be 'eating' when you use conventional cosmetics:

Synthetic Colors: Derived from coal tar, which when injected into lab rats causes cancer. These are typically listed on products as D&C or FD&C.

Diethanolamine and Triethanolamine (DEA and TEA): These two dangerous ingredients are used as emulsifiers, and are known to cause lab rats to develop cancerous tumors. The Cosmetics Review Panel recommends only small amounts; however, small amounts add up over time.

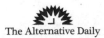

Titanium Dioxide: This is found in concealers, and is noted by the American Cancer Society as being one of the top five most carcinogenic substances on earth. It has been implicated in cancer, asthma, kidney disease, loss of fertility and Alzheimer's. Also found in some vitamins, cheeses, yogurts, fast foods and tomato ketchup, this highly toxic chemical is also fed to animals bred for human consumption.

Heavy Metals: Lead has been found in over 500 brands and shades of lipsticks, and although the FDA says that trace amounts are not dangerous, numerous studies show that lead builds up in the system and is indeed highly dangerous. Metals are also used for color, and many lip glosses contain aluminum compounds.

PVP/VA Copolymer: Bronzers, eye makeup and hair products contain this known toxin. In laboratory settings, rats who ingested PVP intravenously developed tumors.

Petrolatum: This is what we know as petroleum, and is used in many popular moisturizers. It forms a layer on the skin, blocks evaporation and prevents toxins from exiting the pores of our skin.

Triclosan: Found in a number of cosmetics and even toothpastes, it is thought to kill bacteria. It was actually invented to be used as a surgical scrub for medical professionals, not for putting on your face or brushing your teeth.

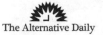

Diazolidinyl Urea: This ingredient is toxic and may release formaldehyde. It is often found in lotions, moisturizers, makeup, sunscreen, shaving products and makeup removers.

Propylene Glycol: This is one of the most commonly used moisture-carrying ingredients in personal care products, and is used in almost all conventional makeup. It has been known to cause serious allergic reactions, including hives, and is also associated with skin conditions such as eczema.

Talc: Talc is also known as hydrous magnesium silicate, which is a toxic ingredient similar to asbestos. It is listed on the Environment Canada Domestic Substance List as "expected to be toxic or harmful," and can be found in eye shadow, face powder and other loose mineral makeup products.

Feed Your Skin Right

Putting any of these toxic chemicals on your skin can actually be worse than eating them. When you eat something, your saliva and stomach help to break it down and get it out of your body. However, when your skin absorbs something it goes straight into the bloodstream without being filtered. Without the necessary enzymes to break them down, these toxins accumulate over time and wreak havoc on the body, accelerating the aging process.

To stay safe, purchase only products that are 100 percent organic. If you cannot pronounce all of the ingredients on the package or do not know what they are, don't feed them to your skin!

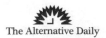

#78 Apple Cider Vinegar for Age Spots

Age spots are skin discolorations found generally on the face, neck or the backs of the hands. Though no two spots are alike, they're generally flat in shape and can range in color from brown or gray to a deeper shade of black in some people.

They're called "liver spots" by some, as holistic practitioners believe that an over-abundance of toxins in the liver or kidneys are a direct cause. Because they usually start popping up in the 40-plus age bracket, they've adopted their most common name, "age spots."

From a scientific standpoint, the spots appear in areas of concentrated melanin production. Melanin is responsible for producing the skin's pigment. Excessive UV exposure can stimulate the overproduction of melanin, and the simple process of aging usually contributes to excessive melanin production, as well. Combine years in the sun and the wear and tear of aging and you've got a recipe for age spots.

Dermatologists will often point patients towards the medical route when it comes to treating age spots. A dermabrasion procedure will essentially sand your skin down to allow for new spot-free growth, or you can opt to burn the top layer of skin off with an acid-based chemical peel. Both procedures are as painful as they sound.

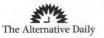
The Alternative Daily

However, there are natural options, and ACV is an excellent one. The sulphur in ACV is effective against signs of aging, including age spots.

HOW TO USE IT: Simply dab a little ACV on age spots each night before you go to bed. If it stings your skin, mix it with a little water. Wash the spot in the morning. Repeat nightly until the spot begins to fade.

Using Apple Cider Vinegar in Your Personal Care Routine

In addition to using organic personal care products, ACV offers a multitude of age defying, toxicity-free benefits and is a great compliment to a natural beauty care regime. Here are just a few of the ways that the whole family can benefit from ACV.

#79 Aftershave

Mix ½ cup of ACV with ½ cup filtered water in a small bottle, and add 20 drops of tea tree oil. Shake the bottle lightly and use after you shave. The mixture will soothe irritated skin and feel refreshing.

#80 Deodorant

Although the smell of ACV is strong, it acts as a powerful deodorant. Rub a little under your arms before you work out, and odor will be a thing of the past.

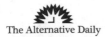

TRY IT: Another way to make your own homemade deodorant using coconut oil, baking soda, arrowroot and essential oils: Simply mix ½ cup of baking soda with ½ cup of arrowroot, and enough melted coconut oil to make a thick paste like glue. Add 20 drops of lavender essential oil for a fresh smell. Store in a small glass jar. Reapply as often as needed during the day.

#81 Hair Rinse

If you wash your hair with conventional shampoo, a residue builds up over time. This can cause your hair to become dull and lifeless. To remove the residue and restore shine and bounce, mix ½ teaspoon of ACV with 1 cup of water and pour onto your hair. If you apply baking soda to your hair first, you will find your hair less frizzy, shinier and healthier. Using this treatment a few times a week also stimulates hair growth and prevents split ends.

Making Your Own Apple Cider Vinegar

Organic, Whole Apple Vinegar Recipe

Although it will take seven months for your vinegar to ferment, the process of making your own is not difficult.

Supplies:

- 10 whole, organic apples of any type
- 1 medium glass bowl
- 1 large glass bowl
- A piece of cheesecloth

Directions:

1. Wash the apples and cut them into quarters.
2. Allow the apples to turn brown in the air.
3. Place in a medium glass bowl and cover with filtered water
4. Cover the bowl with the cheesecloth and leave it in a warm, dark place for six months.
5. After six months you will see a gray-colored scum on the surface of the liquid – this is normal.
6. Strain the liquid through a coffee filter into a larger glass bowl.
7. Cover the bowl with the cheesecloth and let it sit for another four weeks.
8. Pour the vinegar into a glass container and use as desired.

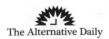

Apple Scraps Recipe

If you are impatient and want your vinegar sooner than seven months, you may want to try this recipe. It is a great way to make use of apple scraps after baking.

Ingredients:

- Wide-mouth jar
- Apple scraps, including cores and peels, from organic apples
- A piece of cheesecloth

Directions:

1. Leave the scraps exposed to air until they turn brown.
2. Add the scraps to the jar and cover with water.
3. Cover the jar with the cheesecloth.
4. Place jar in a warm, dark place.
5. In a few days you will see the contents thicken and a gray scum appear.
6. Allow the apples to ferment for one month.
7. Taste the vinegar – if it is strong enough, strain the liquid. If not, allow it to sit a while longer and then strain.
8. Store your vinegar in a glass container.

The Alternative Daily

Conclusion

Through the years, there have been thousands of reports regarding apple cider vinegar and its health benefits. As you can see from this book, there are many ways that ACV can help you be the healthiest you can be. If you are interested in home and natural therapies, we encourage you to embrace all that ACV has to offer.

"The art of healing comes from nature and not from the physician. Therefore, the physician must start from nature with an open mind." ~Paracelsus

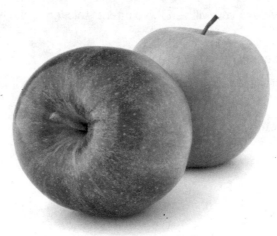

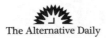

Sources

1 Diabetes Care 27 January, 281-282

2 WebMD, Weight Loss & Diet Plans, Apple Cider Vinegar

3 British Journal of Nutrition May, 95(5):916-924,

4 Bioscience, Biotechnology, and Biochemistry, 65(12) 2690-2694

5 WebMD, Weight Loss & Diet Plans, Apple Cider Vinegar

6 Discover Fit & Health, Health Benefits of Vinegar Overview

7 Vinegar History

8 WiseGeek, What Are the Health-Promoting Properties of Mother of Vinegar

9 WebMD, Healthy Eating & Diet, Apple cider vinegar

10 Discover Fit & Health, How Vinegar Affects Digestion

Effectiveness of malic acid 1% in patients with xerostomia induced by antihypertensive drugs

National Fibromyalgia Association

11 Pet Care with Apple Cider Vinegar

Indian Express Try Apple Cider Vinegar to Cure Digestive Problems

Healthy Healing.com

The Vinegar Institute

Preventative Medicine Research Institute

Effect of a high-molecular-weight component of cranberry on constituents of dental biofilm

BodyEcology.com

Home Remedies Web

Vinegar Ingestion at Bedtime Moderates Waking Glucose Concentrations in Adults With Well-Controlled Type 2 Diabetes

Generation of antitumor active neutral medium-sized alpha-glycan in apple vinegar fermentation

Vinegar: Medicinal Uses and Antiglycemic Effect

Insomnia Linked to Mortality Risk

Cosmetic Ingredient Review

Acne.org

95th Street Dental

Prescription for Nutritional Healing; Phyllis A. Balch

The Illustrated Encyclopedia of Healing Remedies; C. Norman Shealy

The People's Pharmacy Guide to Home and Herbal Remedies; Joe Graedon, MS, Teresa Graedon

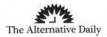

32 Purifying

Apple Cider Vinegar Recipes

That Instantly Unleash Your Well-Being

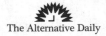

The Alternative Daily

This page intentionally left blank.

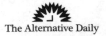

Table of Contents

The Alternative Daily

This page intentionally left blank.

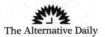

Using Apple Cider Vinegar in Your Diet

Incorporating apple cider vinegar into your diet is easy with these tasty recipes. Just be sure to purchase high-quality, organic, unpasteurized apple cider vinegar that contains mother of vinegar.

#1 Sage and Rosemary Pork Marinade

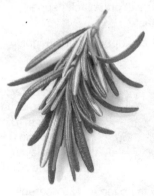

- 1 cup organic apple cider vinegar
- 1/4 cup olive oil
- 1/2 teaspoon coconut crystals
- 1/2 teaspoon fresh pressed garlic
- 1/4 teaspoon sage
- 3 sprigs fresh rosemary

Directions:

Mix the ingredients together in a glass jar and shake well

Apply with a brush

#2 Large Crowd Carrot and Pumpkin Soup

- 4 baking pumpkins, quartered (2 lbs each)
- 4 carrots, peeled and sliced thick
- 6 shallots, sliced thick
- 2 celery stalks, sliced thick
- 4 cloves garlic, minced
- 12 cups vegetable broth
- 1 cup heavy cream
- Olive oil, as needed
- Coconut oil, as needed
- 3/4 teaspoon grated nutmeg
- 1/2 teaspoon cinnamon
- 1 teaspoon fresh sage
- Sea salt and black pepper to taste
- 1/4 cup apple cider vinegar

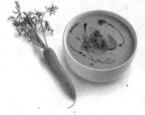

Directions:

Adjust your racks so that one is on the upper third of the oven and one is on the lower third of the oven

Preheat the oven to 425 degrees F

Spread out your pumpkins cut side down on the baking sheet, drizzle with olive oil and sprinkle with sea salt and black pepper

Roast the pumpkins for about 45 minutes, turning occasionally until they are tender and brown

Rotate the baking sheets about halfway through the roasting

Let the pumpkins cool and scoop the flesh out into a bowl

Warm 2 tablespoons of extra virgin coconut oil over medium heat and add the carrots, shallots and celery; season with salt and pepper

Cover the pot and cook until the vegetables soften - stir often

Add the garlic, nutmeg, cinnamon, sage and apple cider vinegar, along with the pumpkin and broth

Cover the pot and bring it to a boil

Cover and simmer on low for about 15 minutes

Puree the soup until it is smooth using a hand immersion blender

Whisk the cream in a bowl until it starts to get thick

Serve the soup warm with the cream on top

This will serve up to 12 people so it is great for a large gathering

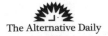

#3 Ginger Refresher

- 2 tablespoons apple cider vinegar
- 4 teaspoons raw stevia
- 1/4 teaspoon ground ginger
- 1 cup filtered water

Directions:

Combine all ingredients in a glass jar and cover.

Refrigerate for at least 2 hours.

Shake well before serving

If you use fresh ginger, strain before drinking

Pour over ice or soda water if desired

#4 Lemon and Honey Detox Tea

- 1 glass filtered warm water (16 ounces)
- 2 tablespoons apple cider vinegar
- 2 tablespoons lemon juice
- 1 teaspoon cinnamon
- 1 teaspoon cayenne pepper
- 1/2 teaspoon raw honey

Directions:

Mix all ingredients together and enjoy

#5 Creamy Oatmeal

- 1 cup rolled organic oats
- 2 cups filtered water
- 2 tablespoons apple cider vinegar
- 1/2 teaspoon Himalayan salt

Directions:

Mix the oats, water and apple cider vinegar in a glass bowl

Cover and let sit for 8 hours (overnight)

Add another cup of filtered water and the salt, stir well

Heat on medium until simmering

Serve with grass fed butter and whole cream

Top with berries of choice

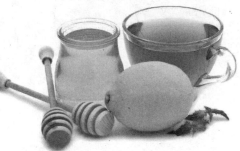

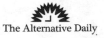

The Alternative Daily

#6 Barbeque Sauce

- 2 cups organic tomato sauce
- 1/2 cup fresh pressed apple juice
- 1/2 cup apple cider vinegar
- 1/2 cup coconut crystals
- 5 tablespoons grass fed butter
- 3 tablespoons paprika
- 2 tablespoons chili powder
- 4 garlic cloves, chopped
- 1/2 onion, finely chopped
- Sea salt to taste
- Touch cayenne pepper

Directions:

Heat the butter in a pot over medium heat for 3 minutes

Add the onions and saute them until they brown

Add the garlic and saute for 2 more minutes

Pour in all of the other ingredients and stir well

Simmer slowly for at least 30 minutes or up to 2 hours

#7 Strawberry Soother

- 8 frozen organic strawberries
- 1/2 cup plain Kefir
- 1/2 cup shredded coconut
- 1/2 teaspoon apple cider vinegar

Directions:

Place all ingredients in a blender and blend until smooth. Optionally, add cinnamon or flax meal.

#8 Marinated Mushrooms

- 12 mushroom caps
- 1/2 cup apple cider vinegar
- 1/4 cup olive oil
- Sea salt and black pepper, to taste
- Cayenne pepper to taste

Directions:

Pour the apple cider vinegar into a large glass jar with a lid

Add the olive oil and shake well

Add the salt, pepper and cayenne and shake again

Add the mushrooms and allow them to soak for 5 hours

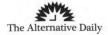

#9 Carrot and Apple Salad

- 1 1/2 tablespoons apple cider vinegar
- 1 small garlic clove, minced
- 1 1/2 tablespoons apple cider vinegar
- 2 cups grated carrots
- 1/2 cup diced red apple
- 1/4 cup sliced green onions
- 1/4 cup fresh parsley
- 1/4 cup chopped dried cranberries
- 1 tablespoon raw honey
- 1 tablespoon olive oil
- 2 cups organic spinach leaves
- Sea salt and black pepper, to taste

Directions:

Mix the apple cider vinegar and garlic in a bowl

Let the mixture sit for 15 minutes

Mix carrots, apple, green onions, parsley and cranberries in a separate large bowl

Pour the honey and oil into the apple cider vinegar mixture and whisk it together

Add the carrot mixture and toss to coat

Season as desired with salt and pepper

Cover the mixture and let it sit for 2 hours to overnight

Serve over a bed of organic spinach

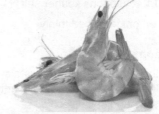

#10 Jake's Famous Steamed Shrimp

- ½ cup apple cider vinegar
- 2 cans of gluten-free light beer
- 1 pound of fresh-caught shrimp, whole
- 2 teaspoons Old Bay seasoning
- Sea salt and black pepper, to taste
- 1 tablespoon grass fed butter

Directions:

Place everything but the shrimp in the stock pot

Add the shrimp when the liquid begins to boil

After about 4-5 minutes, when all the shrimp are pink turn the burner off

Drain the shrimp and enjoy!

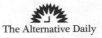

The Alternative Daily

#11 Pickled Red Onions

- 1/2 cup apple cider vinegar
- 1 teaspoon coconut crystals
- 1 1/2 teaspoons kosher salt
- 1 red onion, sliced thinly

Directions:

Whisk the vinegar, coconut crystals and salt together in a small bowl until the crystals and salt dissolve

Place the onion in a clean glass jar

Pour the vinegar over the onions

Let sit at room temperature for 1 hour

Drain the onions

Cover and chill

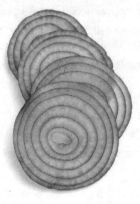

#12 Glazed Buttered Carrots

- 2 pounds medium organic carrots, peeled
- 1 cup apple cider vinegar
- 1/2 cup water
- 2 tablespoons grass fed butter, cut into small pieces
- Sea salt and black pepper, to taste

Directions:

Cut out a piece of wax paper big enough to fit inside a 12-inch heavy skillet

Coat the paper with butter

Cut carrots into 1/2 inch slices

Add to the skillet along with the apple cider vinegar, water, butter, salt and pepper

Cover the carrots with the wax paper, butter side down, and simmer

Lift the paper from time to time to stir the carrots and simmer until the liquid is almost all evaporated (about 40 minutes)

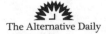

#13 Coconut Onion Soup

- 4 tablespoons grass fed butter
- 3 tablespoons organic coconut oil
- 6 large onions, halved and thinly sliced
- 3 cups chicken broth
- 2 cups apple cider vinegar
- 12 fresh thyme sprigs
- Sea salt and black pepper, to taste
- Chopped thyme, as garnish

Directions:

Melt the butter with the coconut oil in a large stock pot

Saute onions until they are soft and brown (about 20 minutes)

Add the apple cider vinegar, broth and 12 sprigs of thyme

Bring the soup to a boil

Lower the heat and season with sea salt and black pepper

Cook soup for 20 minutes uncovered, then remove thyme sprigs

Serve with chopped thyme and a sprinkle of fresh parmesan cheese

#14 Apple Cider Chutney

- 6 cups organic apple cider
- 1/2 cup apple cider vinegar
- 20 ounces pearl onions, blanched, drained and peeled
- 3/4 cup organic raisins
- 1/4 cup coconut sugar
- 1/4 teaspoon ground cloves
- 1/4 teaspoon nutmeg
- Sea salt and pepper to taste

Directions:

Mix all ingredients together in a large saucepan

Add salt and pepper to taste

Boil for about 30 minutes, stirring occasionally

Serve with roasted grass fed meat or free range poultry

The Alternative Daily

#15 Coconut Honey Dressing

- 2/3 cup organic coconut oil
- 2/3 cup local honey
- 3 tablespoons apple cider vinegar
- Tuscan seasoning, to taste
- Sea salt and pepper, to taste

Directions:

Mix everything but honey together

Gradually whisk honey into the mixture

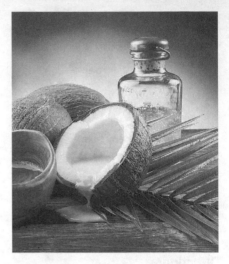

#16 Country Beet Salad

- 2 cups cooked and diced beets (cold)
- 2 cups steamed green beans, cut into halves (cold)
- 2 granny smith apples, diced
- 1 teaspoon coconut oil
- 2 tablespoons apple cider vinegar
- Sea salt and pepper, to taste

Directions:

Toss beets, green beans and apples in a serving bowl

Drizzle with oil and vinegar and toss lightly

Add salt and pepper to taste

#17 Orange and Lemon Salad Dressing

- 1/3 cup fresh squeezed orange juice
- 1/4 cup olive oil
- 1/4 cup apple cider vinegar
- 1/2 teaspoon lemon juice
- 1/2 teaspoon pure honey
- Sprinkle Italian seasoning

Directions:

Combine all ingredients and let sit for one hour before using

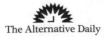

#18 Barbeque Chicken with Sweet and Spicy Glaze

- 1 1/2 cups apple cider vinegar
- 4 teaspoons chili powder
- 2 1/2 teaspoons sea salt
- 1 1/2 teaspoons coconut sugar
- 1 teaspoon cayenne powder
- 1 teaspoon dry mustard
- 1 teaspoon paprika
- 1 teaspoon black pepper
- 1/2 teaspoon cumin
- 4 free range, boneless chicken breasts

Directions:

Combine everything but chicken in a bowl and whisk

Place the chicken in a shallow glass dish and pour the sauce over it; turn chicken to coat evenly

Let sit for 30 minutes

Cook chicken, baste with sauce

#19 Green Smoothie Delight

- 1 large orange, peeled and segmented
- 1/2 large banana, sliced into chunks
- 1/2 avocado
- 5 large frozen strawberries
- 2 cups organic spinach leaves
- 1/3 cup organic Greek yogurt - plain
- 1/2 tablespoon apple cider vinegar
- 1/2 cup ice

Directions:

Place all ingredients in a blender and blend until smooth

#20 Apple Cider Syrup

- 2 cups organic apple cider
- 3/4 cups coconut sugar
- 3 tablespoons grass fed butter
- 2 teaspoons apple cider vinegar

Directions:

Place all ingredients in a saucepan and boil until reduced to about 1 cup

Cool until just warm and serve over homemade ice cream, organic Greek yogurt or organic rice pudding

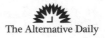

Age-Defying Skin and Body Recipes

Apple cider vinegar contains antifungal, antibacterial and antioxidant powers that can keep you looking and feeling young. Instead of spending a lot of money on commercial personal care products, try these inexpensive, non-toxic alternatives.

#21 Refreshing Foot Soak

Fill a large bowl with warm water and add 1 cup of apple cider vinegar and 1 cup of Epsom salts. Soak your feet for about 20 minutes and pat dry. Follow up with a light coat of hemp oil and slip on some cozy socks. Your feet will be soft and clean.

#22 Green Tea Sugar Face Scrub

Mix 1 teaspoon of apple cider vinegar with 2 teaspoons of cooled, organic green tea, 1 teaspoon of pure local honey and 5 teaspoons of organic brown sugar. Stir thoroughly and apply to your face, rubbing lightly in an upwards and circular motion. Rinse with warm water and pat dry.

#23 Eucalyptus Facial Steam

Mix 2 ounces of ACV with 1 quart of water and add 10 drops of eucalyptus essential oil. Heat the mixture until hot and add a rosemary sprig. Pour into a shallow bowl and lower your head over the bowl (be careful not to touch the water). Cover your head with a towel and breathe in deeply while your skin is refreshed and cleansed. Pat your face with a clean towel and apply an organic skin moisturizer.

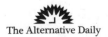

#24 Refreshing Hair Rinse

After using an organic shampoo, nothing makes your scalp feel more refreshed than rinsing it with apple cider vinegar. Add 8 drops of your favorite essential oil, such as lemon, mint or rosemary, to 1/2 cup of apple cider vinegar. Adjust according to length of hair. Spray over hair and let sit for a few minutes, then rinse with warm water.

#25 Dry Hands Soak

Combine 2 cups of warm water with 1 cup of apple cider vinegar and 3 tablespoons of olive oil. Soak dry hands for 10 minutes and pat dry. Follow with a light layer of hemp oil.

#26 Oily Skin Remedy

Combine pure honey, coconut flour and apple cider vinegar to make a paste. Cover your face with the paste and leave on overnight. Rinse in the morning and pat dry. Repeat twice a week to help balance skin.

#27 Super Hand Cleaner

Moisten some cornmeal with apple cider vinegar and use to scrub stains from your hands. Rinse well and pat dry.

#28 All-Over Body Spritz

Mix 1 cup of filtered water with 1/2 cup of apple cider vinegar and 10 drops of clary sage essential oil. Pour the mixture in a spray bottle. Spray a light mist all over your body any time you want to feel refreshed.

The Alternative Daily

Clean Home Recipes

Not only is apple cider vinegar useful for your body, it can also be employed throughout your home.

#29 Good for Everything Cleaner

This cleaner works great for mirrors, windows, sinks and countertops. Combine 1 cup of apple cider vinegar with 2 cups warm water and 6 drops of grapefruit essential oil. Pour into a spray bottle and use to clean mirrors, windows, sinks, countertops and more. Add 2 teaspoons baking soda for really tough jobs.

#30 Wood Paneling Cleaner

To bring out the luster in your wood paneling, mix 1 pint of warm water, 4 tablespoons of apple cider vinegar and 2 tablespoons of olive oil. Pour the mixture into a jar with a lid and shake to mix. Apply with a clean cloth, allowing the solution to soak into wood. Buff with a soft cloth.

#31 Scratch Remover

Make scratches on wood furniture less noticeable. Mix 1 cup of apple cider vinegar with iodine (more iodine for darker wood, more vinegar for lighter wood) in a small jar and use a foam brush to paint over the scratch. Experiment with just the right amounts of vinegar and iodine to cover the scratch.

#32 Faucet Cleaner

To remove hard water buildup and grime from your bathroom or kitchen faucets, simply fill a plastic baggie with apple cider vinegar and add a few drops of lemon essential oil. Tie the baggie over the faucet, securing it with a rubber band. Allow the solution to sit overnight, and rinse in the morning.

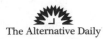

Conclusion

As you embark on your journey to cleanse your body and home, we hope that these recipes will serve as an excellent tool to assist you along the way. Raw apple cider vinegar is truly a gift from nature that is too valuable to pass up. Using it in your diet, personal care regimen and around your home, is a safe and effective way to promote overall health and wellbeing.

"By cleansing your body on a regular basis and eliminating as many toxins as possible from your environment, your body can begin to heal itself, prevent disease, and become stronger and more resilient than you ever dreamed possible!"
~Dr. Edward Group III

The Alternative Daily

2/3 cup of 99% rubbing alcohol
1/3 cup of aloe vera gel
8 to 10 drops essential lavender
vanilla